Living in the Land of Limbo

LIVING
in the Land of Limbo

☙

FICTION AND POETRY
ABOUT FAMILY CAREGIVING

Carol Levine, Editor

VANDERBILT UNIVERSITY PRESS
NASHVILLE

Published 2014 by Vanderbilt University Press
Nashville, Tennessee 37325
All rights reserved
First printing 2014

This book is printed on acid-free paper.
Manufactured in the United States of America

Library of Congress Cataloging-in-Publication Data on file
LC control number 2013034803
LC classification number PS509.C35 L58 2013
Dewey class number 810.8'03561—dc23

ISBN 978-0-8265-1969-6 (hardcover)
ISBN 978-0-8265-1970-2 (paperback)
ISBN 978-0-8265-1971-9 (ebook)

For Howard Lincoln Levine

With love and memories

Contents

PART III
Parents and Sick Children

PART IV
Relatives, Lovers, and Friends

PART V
Paid Caregivers

Acknowledgments

Some books seem to move almost effortlessly from idea to printed page. This is not that sort of book. Over the many years that I collected the selections that appear here (and many others that do not), there were long periods when I felt unable to move forward because of the stresses of caring for my late husband, the exciting but challenging responsibilities of my day job, and the difficulty of seeing how all these pieces that felt so right individually could possibly fit together. Several people made a difference at key points: Michael Ames, Vanderbilt University Press's publisher, helped me shape the book and was always encouraging; my friends Richard and Carole Rifkind greeted my tentative description with enthusiasm and practical suggestions; and John Thornton, my agent who is also an editor and anthologist, was a constant source of advice and support. Fred Courtright handled the complicated task of obtaining permissions, a contribution not usually acknowledged by editors but one that should be. Finally, the Winston Foundation provided a grant that greatly aided in the completion of the book. My children and grandchildren provided ample distraction and much joy.

Living in the Land of Limbo

Introduction: Family Caregivers in Fiction and Poetry

Carol Levine

> The chronically ill often are like those trapped at a frontier, wandering confused in a poorly known border area, waiting desperately to return to their native land. . . . This image should also alert us to the . . . entrance and exit formalities . . . and especially [to] the relatives and friends who press their faces against windows to wave a sad goodbye, who carry sometimes the heaviest baggage, who sit in the same waiting rooms, and who even travel through the same land of limbo, experiencing similar worry, hurt, uncertainty and loss. . . .
>
> —Arthur Kleinman, *The Illness Narratives: Suffering, Healing and the Human Condition* (New York: Basic Books, 1988), p. 183

If birth and death are universal, the experience of caring for someone with a chronic or terminal illness is nearly so. Despite a pervasive myth of family abandonment, most people are accompanied and cared for through illness or disability by relatives, friends, and others close to them. These caregivers—"family" understood broadly—live in the land of limbo. Kleinman, a renowned psychiatrist and anthropologist, has now entered the land of limbo himself, as he cares for his wife who has Alzheimer's disease.[1]

Kleinman located the region of limbo aptly. According to early Christian theologians, "limbo," where innocent souls wander, lies at the border of Hell. Its theological history aside, limbo today means a state of uncertainty, a feeling of being trapped, waiting for events beyond one's control to unfold. What family caregiver has not at some time felt isolated, confined, and unsure of when or where or how the difficult journey will end! It is a journey that most embark on out of love or obligation. And yet there are no maps or GPS systems to guide confused travelers.

In an aging society, when medical miracles save and prolong lives but do not necessarily cure, caregiving is becoming a normative experience. An estimated forty-two million Americans now care for an elderly, disabled, or chronically ill adult. Millions more take care of chronically ill or disabled children. In the past few years, in response to this phenomenon, there has been an outpouring of practical handbooks to give family caregivers tools to perform the medical, financial, and legal tasks they undertake and for which they are so poorly prepared by the medical and social service systems. There are also many first-person narratives by caregivers that describe their own powerful and painful journeys. In addition, many books offer to help caregivers "cope" with tips about wellness, self-help, and spiritual renewal. Finally, there are professional books that are intended to educate doctors, nurses, social workers, and others about the crises faced by their patients' families. These are typically written from a disciplinary perspective such as gerontology, social work, or nursing.

This book about caregiving is different. It is not intended to teach, train, or inspire. It offers no helpful tips about reaching out to others for help or navigating the health care system. It does not encourage policy makers to recognize and support family caregivers in tangible, not just rhetorical, ways. Such books have worthy goals, and I have contributed to many of them.

This book is intended to enrich readers' understanding of family caregiving, whether the reader is a family caregiver, health care or social service professional, relative, or friend. It does this by drawing on a largely untapped resource: the wisdom, wit, and artistry of the creative writers of the past half century.[2] Poets and writers of fiction have much to say about suffering, healing, grief, and the human condition—the essence of caregiving.

There is, of course, a large and growing body of narratives and memoirs about illness and caregiving. Memoirs describe reality, or at least reality as the writer experienced it. Many of the selections in this book are based on personal experiences, but the authors have chosen to transcend reality by turning it into art. In Lorrie Moore's story "People Like That Are the Only People Here," the Mother, a writer, reflects after her baby's cancer surgery, "How can it be described? How can any of it be described? The trip and the story of the trip are always two different things."

Rochelle Almeida in her study of mourning says, "I believe that short fiction enables the writer and the reader to distill the very essence of personal loss by boiling human emotion down to the barest bones and saying it all most eloquently."[3]

Novelist Amy Tan says, "In writing, I always try to draw upon the emotional truth of my past experiences but never on the actual factual truth. I alter the details while trying to retain the sensual impact. This it seems to me is what fiction does and what makes it often more effective than straight biography or memoir."[4]

Similarly, Joyce Carol Oates, who has written both a memoir (*A Widow's Story*) and short stories in which widows are the main characters (*Sourland*), responded to Jeffrey Brown's question on *PBS NewsHour*: "Is fiction better for some things—and nonfiction for others?" by stating "Yes, fiction is much better for some things, definitely. The sort of thing that I want to do is to strike a resonant chord of universality in other people, which is best done by fiction."[5]

One further distinction: poetry and fiction are often more concerned with the body and bodily functions than memoirs. Many of the selections in this volume are quite explicit about this aspect of caregiving. Rick Moody's description of a son bathing his debilitated mother in "Whosoever" might seem inappropriate in a memoir but provides an extraordinary insight into this common experience precisely because it is fiction.

THE STORY BEHIND THE STORIES

Anthologies by their very nature are reflections of the editor's viewpoint. I can imagine a reader asking, "From all the stories and poems in all the books and journals from the past fifty years, why did you pick these?" And "Why didn't you go back further into history and include Edith Wharton's *Ethan Frome* or a Chekhov story?" Fair questions that deserve answers. The second question is easy. I wanted the selections to be contemporary so that readers would not have to delve further to understand the language or the context. The first question takes a little more explaining. My professional work in the field of caregiving over the past twenty years sits squarely in nonfiction. Apart from a few short essays about my experiences caring for my late husband Howard, who suffered a traumatic brain injury in an automobile accident and was left quadriplegic, I have stayed close to the world of facts and research findings and policy analysis. Write a poem? Never! A short story? Wouldn't know how. But in the seventeen years I cared for Howard at home, I found myself turning more and more to poetry and short fiction as a source of solace and a way to gain meaning from what sometimes seemed bereft of meaning. To my surprise, many of the stories were funny, or at least captured the absurdity of some aspects of caregiving.

I found I learned more about myself and my situation from these unlikely sources than from the more conventional coping literature. And I learned much more about caregivers who are different from me and face different challenges. In fact, the more specific the context, the more I learned about the individuals in the story. The Japanese-American mother in Julie Otsuka's story "Diem Perdidi" recalls her childhood in an internment camp in World War II but cannot remember her daughter's name. The story was moving both as a tale of dementia and as a reminder of the persistence of memory.

This book is a selection of some of the pieces I read when I was unable to sleep, alert for my husband's call, and when I was traveling for work and worried about him even though he was well taken care of. And after he died, I continued to collect possible selections. Some I came across randomly, others were suggested to me by colleagues. Interestingly, when I described this project to colleagues, stressing that I was looking for short stories and poems, they immediately suggested memoirs. That genre is certainly alive and well, and perhaps this anthology will bring an alternative to more readers.

I was drawn to writing that had literary merit, not just an interesting character or a difficult situation. So this anthology contains the spare voices of W. S. Merwin and Raymond Carver, the exquisitely convoluted sentences of Rick Moody, and the dreamlike descriptions of Julie Otsuka.

I did not choose the selections because they portray caregivers in either a positive or negative light. The caregivers in these stories and poems are, variously, ambivalent, selfish, angry, self-sacrificing, strong, resourceful, fallible—in other words, human. Nor did I look for examples of uncaring health care professionals, though they showed up fairly frequently on their own. The case worker in Allegra Goodman's story "The Closet," for example, agrees that Evelyn's sister Lily is mentally ill but says that Lily's decision to live in a closet is simply a "lifestyle choice." The doctors in Lorrie Moore's story are portrayed with all their blunt doctor-speak: "We can't tell until it [her baby's kidney] is in the bucket." On the other hand, Celia, the main character in Ann Harleman's story "Thoreau's Laundry," is both a technician who makes facial prostheses for injured patients and a family caregiver. For the most part, however, professionals don't play much of a role in these selections. As in life, they come and go, while caregiving goes on and on.

ORGANIZATION OF THE BOOK

The book is divided into five sections, each with a short introduction, based on the relationship of the caregiver to the person needing assistance: children of aging parents; husbands and wives; parents and sick children (including adult children); relatives, lovers, and friends; and paid caregivers. I was pleased to be able to include a few selections in this last category, which does not generally get much attention in either memoirs or fiction. Not surprisingly, the first two categories—children caring for aging parents and husbands and wives—are mostly concerned with dementia, and the fourth—relatives, lovers and friends—contains stories and a poem about people with HIV/AIDS. There are also stories about mental illness and two poems about cancer. In some cases the disease is not specified. The important aspect of each piece to me was not the diagnosis but the relationship of the people involved and how illness affected them.

What had to be left out? There are several excellent treatments of caregiving in novels and plays, such as Walter Mosely's novel *The Last Days of*

Ptolemy Gray, Michael Ignatieff's novel *Scar Tissue*, and Terrence McNally's play, *Love! Valour! Compassion!* They were excluded from this edition because it would be unwieldy to explain the context of an excerpt. Other selections were not available because of permission requirements. Please let me know if you have a favorite story or poem (not memoir) that might be included in another edition.

HOW TO USE THIS BOOK

Health care professionals such as doctors, nurses, and social workers are coming into contact more and more often with family caregivers and seek understanding of their roles and problems. Gerontologists and other academic researchers are focusing on aging and disabilities, and increasingly that includes the family members of their primary subjects. The overall category of "humanities and medicine" is taught in some form in most professional schools. Narrative medicine is a growing subdivision of the humanities curriculum. These stories and poems can add to the literature used in these classes.

Leaders of support groups for caregivers can select from these stories and poems to start a discussion about the caregivers' reactions with questions like, "Do you see yourself in the characters?" "Do you judge the characters?" "What seems vivid and real and what seems arbitrary?"

And for caregivers who can't sleep or who are away from home or who just want a new perspective on their lives, I hope they find in this book new ways to map their journey out of limbo into the light.

NOTES

1. Arthur Kleinman, "Caregiving: The Odyssey of Becoming More Human," *Lancet* 373, no. 9660 (Jan. 2009): 292–293, doi: 10.1016/S0140-6736(09)60087-8.
2. There are two partial exceptions. Nell Casey's book, *An Uncertain Inheritance: Writers on Caring for Family* (New York: Morrow, 2007) is a collection of memoirs by well-known writers. *Stories of Family Caregiving: Reconsiderations of Theory, Literature, and Life*, edited by Suzanne Poirier and Lioness Ayres (Indianapolis: Center Nursing Publishing, 2002), discusses both fiction (mostly novels) and nonfiction and provides a bibliography. Only brief quotes from the literature are in the text.
3. Rochelle Almeida, *The Politics of Mourning* (Madison, NJ: Fairleigh Dickinson University Press, 2004), 15.
4. Molly Giles, "Author Q&A: A Conversation with Amy Tan," Random House Publishing Group, accessed Nov. 7, 2013, *www.randomhouse.com/rhpg//rc/library/display.pperl?isbn=9780345457370&view=qa*
5. "Joyce Carol Oates on 'Absurdity' of Widowhood," *PBS NewsHour*, aired Feb. 3, 2011. *video.pbs.org/program/newshour*

PART I
Children of Aging Parents

The typical family caregiver—as portrayed over and over in the media—is a forty-something woman taking care of a parent (or two) who has young or teenage children and a full-time job. Through it all she gives credit to her patient husband and says it is a blessing to take care of her beloved parent (or two). This scenario is, for many people, the way things are, ever were, and ever should be.

Certainly such situations exist. But this picture fails to capture the reality of many caregivers' lives. With the aging of American society and advances in health care technology, more people with serious chronic illnesses, especially dementia, are living longer, increasing the extent and intensity of care and support needed. Caregiving takes place over years, not months, and family members' chronic conditions require more and more medical interventions and a tote bag full of medications. The "sick room" of nineteenth and early twentieth century stories today looks more like a hospital room than a bedroom.

To take one example: Julia Stephen, Virginia Woolf's mother, was a nurse. In 1883 she wrote a guide called "Notes from Sick Rooms." Given the complexity of home care today, it is disconcerting to read Stephen's extensive comments about the persistent problem of nothing less than crumbs in the bed. While crumbs in the bed may not rate high on the list of today's caregivers' worries, much of caregiving involves just that kind of mundane task, part of the range of high- and low-tech tasks that characterize caregiving today. Tedium is interrupted by crisis. And through it all, the caregiver does not know when one will give way to the other.

In addition to advancing ages, the population is also becoming more diverse. As a result of these and other societal changes, the picture of family caregiving today is more a mosaic than a single image. Caregivers today are almost as likely to be men as women (although women still carry the heaviest loads), they come from all ethnic groups, and they react differently to the responsibilities thrust upon them as parents age.

The stories in this section illustrate that diversity. In "Diem Perdidi" (I have lost the day), Julie Otsuka describes an aging parent's deterioration into full-blown dementia. In a sly reference to the standard questions a doctor may ask an older patient, the story begins, "She remembers her name. She remembers the name of the president. She remembers the name of the president's dog. . . ." But "She does not remember what she ate for dinner last night, or when she last took her medicine." Nor does she remember the daughter/narrator's name. This careful cataloging of what "she" does and does not remember is suffused with her memories of being a child interned with her Japanese-American family in World War II.

Rick Moody's story "Whosoever: The Language of Mothers and Sons" is almost a Biblical incantation. This story is the first chapter of Moody's 1996 novel "Purple America," which takes place in suburban Connecticut. The son who returns home without realizing how disabled his mother has become gives her a bath. Standard caregiving task, but Moody turns it into a mystical experience. "Whosoever knows the folds and complexities of his own mother's body, *he shall never die.*"

In the third story in this section, "The Third Dumpster," by Gish Jen, two Chinese-American sons try to fix up an old house for their parents, who have rejected assisted living because of the Western food. They scoff, "*Lamb chops! Salad!*" "Their parents were *Chinese, end of story,* as Morehouse [one of the sons] liked to say." These differences in opinion between parents and children about where to live or who should provide care are familiar to many caregivers.

Two of the poems in this section continue the imagery of water and bathing in Moody's story. "Water" by Li-Young Lee has many images of water, but the poem is mainly about his father: "Water has invaded my father's / heart, swollen, heavy, / twice as large. Bloated / liver. Bloated legs." He gently washes his father's feet, testing the water with his wrist. He knows that water will kill his father, even as water brought him freedom from torture in Indonesia to America. In "Lucky" by Tony Hoagland, again a son bathes his mother, now a "childish skeleton." His act of devotion is also an act of revenge, against an "old enemy." Hoagland has described this poem as being "American" in its "merciless candor."[1]

Two other poems are about sons and fathers. The spare language in David Mason's poem "Fathers and Sons" conceals the emotion a son feels as he helps his father go to the toilet. "Yesterday" by W. S. Merwin is about the relationships between two fathers and sons—the friend he meets who describes a visit to his father, and the memories this conversation evokes about the poet's own father. The friend's distant relationship with his father is evoked simply yet powerfully.

Robert Pinsky's "Ode to Meaning" is a dense and complicated poem with many classical allusions. Its link to caregiving is not immediately apparent. It is, as the title says, an ode, a hymn of praise. In it Pinsky refers to his mother's fall on her head. He says, "For years afterward, she had various symptoms that made the household somewhat chaotic. Meaning became a prized rarity. . . ." The opposite of meaning, he says, "is not necessarily meaninglessness: it might be the arbitrary."[2] The third stanza, where the words appear in alphabetical order, illustrates this.

Finally, this section ends with two poems about sons and mothers. James Dickey, in "Buckdancer's Choice," describes his mother in her invalid bed, warbling the thousand variations of a minstrel song. Both she and the classic buck-and-wing men are dying out. Raymond Carver conveys a son's frustration with his mother's failing memory and constant neediness in his poem "Where the Groceries Went." On the phone he reminds her that she has plenty of food in the house. But she is "afraid of everything." And while he feels he is trying to be a good son, she is bitter. She says, that if only he would help her, then he could go back to "whatever / it was that was so important / I had to take the trouble / to bring you into this world."

NOTES

1. Brian Brodeur, "Tony Hoagland," *How a Poem Happens: Contemporary Poets Discuss the Making of Poems* (blog), Nov. 5, 2009, *howapoemhappens. blogspot.com/2009/11/tony-hoagland.html*
2. Robert Pinsky, "Contributors' Notes and Comments," in *The Best American Poetry 1998*, ed. David Lehman and John Hollander (New York: Scribner, 1998), 317–318.

1

Diem Perdidi

❧ Julie Otsuka

She remembers her name. She remembers the name of the president. She remembers the name of the president's dog. She remembers what city she lives in. And on which street. And in which house. *The one with the big olive tree where the road takes a turn.* She remembers what year it is. She remembers the season. She remembers the day on which you were born. She remembers the daughter who was born before you—*She had your father's nose, that was the first thing I noticed about her*—but she does not remember that daughter's name. She remembers the name of the man she did not marry—Frank—and she keeps his letters in a drawer by her bed. She remembers that you once had a husband but she refuses to remember your ex-husband's name. *That man*, she calls him.

She does not remember how she got the bruises on her arms or going for a walk with you earlier this morning. She does not remember bending over, during that walk, and plucking a flower from a neighbour's front yard and slipping it into her hair. *Maybe your father will kiss me now.* She does not remember what she ate for dinner last night, or when she last took her medicine. She does not remember to drink enough water. She does not remember to comb her hair.

She remembers the rows of dried persimmons that once hung from the eaves of her mother's house in Berkeley. *They were the most beautiful shade of orange.* She remembers that your father loves peaches. She remembers that every Sunday morning, at ten, he takes her for a drive down to the sea in the brown car. She remembers that every evening, right before the eight o'clock news, he sets out two fortune cookies on a paper plate and announces to her that they are having a party. She remembers that on Mondays he comes home from the college at four, and if he is even five minutes late she goes out to the gate and begins to wait for him. She remembers which bedroom is hers and which is his. She remembers that the bedroom

---

"Diem Perdidi" was first published in *Granta*. Reprinted by permission of Julie Otsuka, Inc. and Aragi, Inc.

that is now hers was once yours. She remembers that it wasn't always like this.

She remembers the first line of the song, "How High the Moon." She remembers the Pledge of Allegiance. She remembers her Social Security number. She remembers her best friend Jean's telephone number even though Jean has been dead for six years. She remembers that Margaret is dead. She remembers that Betty is dead. She remembers that Grace has stopped calling. She remembers that her own mother died nine years ago, while spading the soil in her garden, and she misses her more and more every day. *It doesn't go away.* She remembers the number assigned to her family by the government right after the start of the war. *13611.* She remembers being sent away to the desert with her mother and brother during the fifth month of that war and taking her first ride on a train. She remembers the day they came home. *September 9, 1945.* She remembers the sound of the wind hissing through the sagebrush. She remembers the scorpions and red ants. She remembers the taste of dust.

Whenever you stop by to see her she remembers to give you a big hug, and you are always surprised at her strength. She remembers to give you a kiss every time you leave. She remembers to tell you, at the end of every phone call, that the FBI will check up on you again soon. She remembers to ask you if you would like her to iron your blouse for you before you go out on a date. She remembers to smooth down your skirt. *Don't give it all away.* She remembers to brush aside a wayward strand of your hair. She does not remember eating lunch with you twenty minutes ago and suggests that you go out to Marie Callender's for sandwiches and pie. She does not remember that she herself once used to make the most beautiful pies with perfectly fluted crusts. She does not remember how to iron your blouse for you or when she began to forget. *Something's changed.* She does not remember what she is supposed to do next.

She remembers that the daughter who was born before you lived for half an hour and then died. *She looked perfect from the outside.* She remembers her mother telling her, more than once, *Don't you ever let anyone see you cry.* She remembers giving you your first bath on your third day in the world. She remembers that you were a very fat baby. She remembers that your first word was *No.* She remembers picking apples in a field with Frank many years ago in the rain. *It was the best day of my life.* She remembers that the first time she met him she was so nervous she forgot her own address. She remembers wearing too much lipstick. She remembers not sleeping for days.

When you drive past Hesse Park, she remembers being asked to leave her exercise class by her teacher after being in that class for more than ten years. *I shouldn't have talked so much.* She remembers touching her toes and doing windmills and jumping jacks on the freshly mown grass. She remembers being the highest kicker in her class. She does not remember how to use the "new" coffee maker, which is now three years old, because it was bought after she began to forget. She does not remember asking your father, ten minutes ago, if today is Sunday, or if it is time to go for her ride. She does not remember where she last put her sweater or how long she has been sitting in her chair. She does not always remember how to get out of that chair, and so you gently push down on the footrest and offer her your hand, which she does not always remember to take. *Go away*, she sometimes says. Other times, she just says, *I'm stuck*. She does not remember saying to you, the other night, right after your father left the room, *He loves me more than I love him*. She does not remember saying to you, a moment later, *I can hardly wait until he comes back*.

She remembers that when your father was courting her he was always on time. She remembers thinking that he had a nice smile. *He still does*. She remembers that when they first met he was engaged to another woman. She remembers that that other woman was white. She remembers that that other woman's parents did not want their daughter to marry a man who looked like the gardener. She remembers that the winters were colder back then, and that there were days on which you actually had to put on a coat and scarf. She remembers her mother bowing her head every morning at the altar and offering her ancestors a bowl of hot rice. She remembers the smell of incense and pickled cabbage in the kitchen. She remembers that her father always wore nice shoes. She remembers that the night the FBI came for him, he and her mother had just had another big fight. She remembers not seeing him again until after the end of the war.

She does not always remember to trim her toenails, and when you soak her feet in the bucket of warm water she closes her eyes and leans back in her chair and reaches out for your hand. *Don't give up on me*. She does not remember how to tie her shoelaces, or fasten the hooks on her bra. She does not remember that she has been wearing her favourite blue blouse for five days in a row. She does not remember your age. *Just wait till you have children of your own*, she says to you, even though you are now too old to do so.

She remembers that after the first girl was born and then died, she sat in the yard for days, just staring at the roses by the pond. *I didn't know what else to do*. She remembers that when you were born you, too, had your father's long nose. *It was as if I'd given birth to the same girl twice*. She remembers that you are a Taurus. She remembers that your birthstone is green. She remembers to read you your horoscope from the newspaper whenever you come over to see her. *Someone you were once very close to may soon reappear in your life*. She does not remember reading you that same horoscope five minutes ago or going to the doctor with you last week after you discovered a bump on the back of her head. *I think I fell.* She does not remember telling the doctor that you are no longer married, or giving him your number and asking him to please call. She does not remember leaning over and whispering to you, the moment he stepped out of the room, *I think he'll do.*

She remembers another doctor asking her, fifty years ago, minutes after the first girl was born and then died, if she wanted to donate the baby's body to science. *He said she had a very unusual heart.* She remembers being in labour for thirty-two hours. She remembers being too tired to think. *So I told him yes.* She remembers driving home from the hospital in the sky-blue Chevy with your father and neither one of them saying a word. She remembers knowing she'd made a big mistake. She does not remember what happened to the baby's body and worries that it might be stuck in a jar. She does not remember why they didn't just bury her. *I wish she were under a tree.* She remembers wanting to bring her flowers every day.

She remembers that even as a young girl you said you did not want to have children. She remembers that you hated wearing dresses. She remembers that you never played with dolls. She remembers that the first time you bled you were thirteen years old and wearing bright yellow pants. She remembers that your childhood dog was named Shiro. She remembers that you once had a cat named Gasoline. She remembers that you had two turtles named Turtle. She remembers that the first time she and your father took you to Japan to meet his family you were eighteen months old and just beginning to speak. She remembers leaving you with his mother in the tiny silkworm village in the mountains while she and your father travelled across the island for ten days. *I worried about you the whole time.* She remembers that when they came back you did not know who she was and that for many days afterwards you would not speak to her, you would only whisper in her ear.

She remembers that the year you turned five you refused to leave the house without tapping the door frame three times. She remembers that you had a habit of clicking your teeth repeatedly, which drove her up the wall. She remembers that you could not stand it when different-coloured foods were touching on the plate. *Everything had to be just so.* She remembers trying to teach you to read before you were ready. She remembers taking you to Newberry's to pick out patterns and fabric and teaching you how to sew. She remembers that every night, after dinner, you would sit down next to her at the kitchen table and hand her the bobby pins one by one as she set the curlers in her hair. She remembers that this was her favourite part of the day. *I wanted to be with you all the time.*

She remembers that you were conceived on the first try. She remembers that your brother was conceived on the first try. She remembers that your other brother was conceived on the second try. *We must not have been paying attention.* She remembers that a palm reader once told her that she would never be able to bear children because her uterus was tipped the wrong way. She remembers that a blind fortune-teller once told her that she had been a man in her past life, and that Frank had been her sister. She remembers that everything she remembers is not necessarily true. She remembers the horse-drawn garbage carts on Ashby, her first pair of crepesoled shoes, scattered flowers by the side of the road. She remembers that the sound of Frank's voice always made her feel calmer. She remembers that every time they parted he turned around and watched her walk away. She remembers that the first time he asked her to marry him she told him she wasn't ready. She remembers that the second time she said she wanted to wait until she was finished with school. She remembers walking along the water with him one warm summer evening on the boardwalk and being so happy she could not remember her own name. She remembers not knowing that it wouldn't be like this with any of the others. She remembers thinking she had all the time in the world.

She does not remember the names of the flowers in the yard whose names she has known for years. *Roses? Daffodils? Immortelles?* She does not remember that today is Sunday, and she has already gone for her ride. She does not remember to call you, even though she always says that she will. She remembers how to play "Clair de Lune" on the piano. She remembers how to play "Chopsticks" and scales. She remembers not to talk to telemarketers when they call on the telephone. *We're not interested.* She remembers her grammar. *Just between you and me.* She remembers her manners. She remembers to say thank you and please. She remembers to wipe herself every time she uses the toilet. She remembers to flush. She remembers to turn her wedding ring around whenever she pulls on her silk stockings. She remembers to reapply her lipstick every time she leaves the house. She remembers to put on her anti-wrinkle cream every night before climbing into bed. *It works while you sleep.* In the morning, when she wakes, she remembers her dreams. *I was walking through a forest. I was swimming in a river. I was looking for Frank in a city I did not know and no one would tell me where he was.*

On Halloween day, she remembers to ask you if you are going out trick-or-treating. She remembers that your father hates pumpkin. *It's all he ate in Japan during the war.* She remembers listening to him pray, every night, when they first got married, that he would be the one to die first. She remembers playing marbles on a dirt floor in the desert with her brother and listening to the couple at night on the other side of the wall. *They were at it all the time.* She remembers the box of chocolates you brought back to her after your honeymoon in Paris. "But will it last?" you asked her. She remembers her own mother telling her, "The moment you fall in love with someone, you are lost."

She remembers that when her father came back after the war he and her mother fought even more than they had before. She remembers that he would spend entire days shopping for shoes in San Francisco while her mother scrubbed other people's floors. She remembers that some nights he would walk around the block three times before coming into the house. She remembers that one night he did not come in at all. She remembers that when your own husband left you, five years ago, you broke out in hives all over your body for weeks. She remembers thinking he was trouble the moment she met him. *A mother knows.* She remembers keeping that thought to herself. *I had to let you make your own mistakes.*

She remembers that, of her three children, you were the most delightful to be with. She remembers that your younger brother was so quiet she sometimes forgot he was there. *He was like a dream.* She remembers that her own brother refused to carry anything with him on to the train except for his rubber toy truck. *He wouldn't let me touch it.* She remembers her mother killing all the chickens in the yard the day before they left. She remembers her fifth-grade teacher, Mr. Martello, asking her to stand up in front of the class so everyone could tell her goodbye. She remembers being given a silver heart pendant by her next-door neighbour, Elaine Crowley, who promised to write but never did. She remembers losing that pendant on the train and being so angry she wanted to cry. *It was my first piece of jewellery.*

She remembers that one month after Frank joined the Air Force he suddenly stopped writing her letters. She remembers worrying that he'd been shot down over Korea or taken hostage by guerrillas in the jungle. She remembers thinking about him every minute of the day. *I thought I was losing my mind.* She remembers learning from a friend one night that he had fallen in love with somebody else. She remembers asking your father the next day to marry her. *"Shall we go get the ring?"* I said to him. She remembers telling him, *"It's time."*

When you take her to the supermarket she remembers that coffee is Aisle Two. She remembers that Aisle Three is milk. She remembers the name of the cashier in the express lane who always gives her a big hug. *Diane.* She remembers the name of the girl at the flower stand who always gives her a single broken-stemmed rose. She remembers that the man behind the meat counter is Big Lou. "Well, hello, gorgeous," he says to her. She does not remember where her purse is, and begins to panic until you remind her that she has left it at home. *I don't feel like myself without it.* She does not remember asking the man in line behind her whether or not he was married. She does not remember him telling her, rudely, that he was not. She does not remember staring at the old woman in the wheelchair by the melons and whispering to you, *I hope I never end up like that.* She remembers that the huge mimosa tree that once stood next to the cart corral in the parking lot is no longer there. *Nothing stays the same.* She remembers that she was once a very good driver. She remembers failing her last driver's test three times in a row. *I couldn't remember any of the rules.* She remembers that the day after her father left them her mother sprinkled little piles of salt in the corner of every room to purify the house. She remembers that they never spoke of him again.

She does not remember asking your father, when he comes home from the pharmacy, what took him so long, or whom he talked to, or whether or not the pharmacist was pretty. She does not always remember his name. She remembers graduating from high school with high honours in Latin. She remembers how to say, "I came, I saw, I conquered." *Vini, vidi, vici.* She remembers how to say, "I have lost the day." *Diem perdidi.* She remembers the words for "I'm sorry" in Japanese, which you have not heard her utter in years. She remembers the words for "rice" and "toilet." She remembers the words for "Wait." *Chotto matte kudasai.* She remembers that a white-snake dream will bring you good luck. She remembers that it is bad luck to pick up a dropped comb. She remembers that you should never run to a funeral. She remembers that you shout the truth down into a well.

She remembers going to work, like her mother, for the rich white ladies up in the hills. She remembers Mrs. Tindall, who insisted on eating lunch with her every day in the kitchen instead of just leaving her alone. She remembers Mrs. Edward deVries, who fired her after one day. *"Who taught you how to iron?" she asked me.* She remembers that Mrs. Cavanaugh would not let her go home on Saturdays until she had baked an apple pie. She remembers Mrs. Cavanaugh's husband, Arthur, who liked to put his hand on her knee. She remembers that he sometimes gave her money. She remembers that she never refused. She remembers once stealing a silver candlestick from a cupboard but she cannot remember whose it was. She remembers that they never missed it. She remembers using the same napkin for three days in a row. She remembers that today is Sunday, which six days out of seven is not true.

When you bring home the man you hope will become your next husband, she remembers to take his jacket. She remembers to offer him coffee. She remembers to offer him cake. She remembers to thank him for the roses. *So you like her?* she asks him. She remembers to ask him his name. *She's my firstborn, you know.* She remembers, five minutes later, that she has already forgotten his name, and asks him again what it is. *That's my brother's name,* she tells him. She does not remember talking to her brother on the phone earlier that morning—*He promised me he'd call*—or going for a walk with you in the park. She does not remember how to make coffee. She does not remember how to serve cake.

She remembers sitting next to her brother many years ago on a train to the desert and fighting about who got to lie down on the seat. She remembers hot white sand, the wind on the water, someone's voice telling her, *Hush, it's all right*. She remembers where she was the day the men landed on the moon. She remembers the day they learned that Japan had lost the war. *It was the only time I ever saw my mother cry*. She remembers the day she learned that Frank had married somebody else. *I read about it in the paper*. She remembers the letter she got from him not long after, asking if he could please see her. *He said he'd made a mistake*. She remembers writing him back, "It's too late." She remembers marrying your father on an unusually warm day in December. She remembers having their first fight, three months later, in March. *I threw a chair*. She remembers that he comes home from the college every Monday at four. She remembers that she is forgetting. She remembers less and less every day.

When you ask her your name, she does not remember what it is. *Ask your father. He'll know*. She does not remember the name of the president. She does not remember the name of the president's dog. She does not remember the season. She does not remember the day or the year. She remembers the little house on San Luis Avenue that she first lived in with your father. She remembers her mother leaning over the bed she once shared with her brother and kissing the two of them goodnight. She remembers that as soon as the first girl was born she knew that something was wrong. *She didn't cry*. She remembers holding the baby in her arms and watching her go to sleep for the first and last time in her life. She remembers that they never buried her. She remembers that they did not give her a name. She remembers that the baby had perfect fingernails and a very unusual heart. She remembers that she had your father's long nose. She remembers knowing at once that she was his. She remembers beginning to bleed two days later when she came home from the hospital. She remembers your father catching her in the bathroom as she began to fall. She remembers a desert sky at sunset. *It was the most beautiful shade of orange*. She remembers scorpions and red ants. She remembers the taste of dust. She remembers once loving someone more than anyone else. She remembers giving birth to the same girl twice. She remembers that today is Sunday, and it is time to go for her ride, and so she picks up her purse and puts on her lipstick and goes out to wait for your father in the car.

2

Whosoever: The Language
of Mothers and Sons

✑ Rick Moody

Whosoever knows the folds and complexities of his own mother's body, *he shall never die*. Whosoever knows the latitudes of his mother's body, whosoever has taken her into his arms and immersed her baptismally in the first-floor tub, lifting one of her alabaster legs and then the other over its lip, whosoever has bathed her with Woolworth's soaps in sample sizes, twisted the creaky taps and tested the water on the inside of his wrist, and shovelled a couple of tablespoons of rose bath salts under the billowing faucet, marveling at their vermillion color, who has bent by hand her sclerotic limbs, as if reassuring himself about the condition of a hinge, and has kissed her on the part that separates the lobes of her white hair, cooed her name while soaping underneath the breast where he was once fed, breathed the acrid and dispiriting stench of her body while scrubbing the greater part of this smell away, pushed her discarded bra and oversized panties (scattered on the tile floor behind him) to one side, away from the water sloshing occasionally over the edge of the tub and choking the runoff drain, who has wiped stalactites of drool from her mouth with a moistened violet washcloth, swept back the annoying violet shower curtain in order to lift up his stick-figure mother and bathe her ass, where a sweet and infantile shit sometimes collects, causing her both discomfort and shame, who has angrily manhandled the dial on the bathroom radio (balanced on the toilet tank) with one wet hand in an effort to find a college station that blasts only compact-disc recordings of train accidents and large-scale construction operations, selecting at last the drummers of Burundi on WUCN knowing full well that his mother can brook only the music of Tin Pan Alley and certain classics, and who has then reacted guiltily at his own selfishness and tuned to some "lite" AM station featuring the greatest hits of swing, whosoever has noticed in the course of his mission the ripe light of early

November as it is played out on the bathroom wall where one of those plug-in electric candles with plastic base is the only source of illumination, and has waited in this half-light while his mother takes her last bodily pleasure—her useless body floating in the warm, humid, even lapping of rose-scented bathwater, a water which in spite of its pleasures occasionally causes transient scotoma, ataxia, difficulty swallowing, deafness, and other temporary dysfunctions consistent with her ailment—who has looked nonetheless at his pacific mom's face in that water and known, in a New Age kind of way, the face he had before he was born, and who has wept over his mother's condition while bathing her, silently weeping, without words or expressions of pity or any nose-blowing or -honking, just weeping for a second like a ninny, and who has thereafter recovered quickly and forcefully from despair, formulating a simple gratitude from the fact that *he still has a mother*, but who has nonetheless wondered at the kind of astral justice that has immobilized her thus, whosoever has then wished that the bath was over already so that he could go and drink too much at a local bar, a bar where he will encounter the citizens of this his *home town*, a bar where he will see his cronies from high school, those who never left, those who have stayed to become civic boosters, those who have sent kids to the same day school they themselves attended thirty years before, who has looked at his watch and yawned, while wondering how long he has to let his mother soak, who soaped his mother a second time, to be sure that every cranny is disinfected, that every particle of dirt, every speck of grime, is eliminated, who stepped into a draining tub to hoist his mother from it, as if he were hoisting a drenched parachute from a streambed, who has balanced her on the closed toilet seat so that he might dry her with a towel of decadent thickness (purple), who has sniffed, lightly, undetectably, the surface of her skin as he dries her, who has refused to put his mother's spectacles on her face just now, as he has in the past when conscripted into bathing her, as he ought to do now, though in all likelihood she can only make out a few blurry shapes anyway (at least until the cooling of her insulted central nervous system), who has wished to prolong this additional disability, however, because when she is totally blind in addition to being damn near quadriplegic she faces up to the fact that her orienting skills are minimal, whosoever has slipped his mother's undergarment about her legs and checked along the way the dainty hairless passage into her vulva one more time, because he can't resist the opportunity here for *knowledge*, who has gagged briefly at his own forwardness, who has strapped his mother's bra onto her and slipped a housedress over her head, getting first one arm and then the other tangled in the neck hole, who has reached for and then pulled the plug on the radio because the song playing on it is too sad, some terribly sad jazz ballad with muted trumpet, who has put slippers on his mother's feet, left and then right, fiddling with her toes briefly first, simply to see if there is any sensation there, because her wasting disease is characterized by periods in which *some* feeling or sensation suddenly returns to affected extremities (though never all sensation), and likewise periods in which sensation is precipitously *snuffed out*, who has noted the complete lack of response in his mother when he pinches her big toe, and who has noted this response calmly, who has now finally set his mother's glasses on her nose and adjusted the stems to make sure they are settled comfortably on her ears, who has kissed her a second time where her disordered hair is thinnest, who has taken her now fully into his arms to carry her to the wheelchair in the doorway, whosoever has said to his wasting mom while stuttering mildly out of generalized anxiety and because of insufficient pause for the inflow and outflow of breath, *Hey, Mom, you look p-p-p-p-p-pretty fabulous t-t-tonight, you look like a million b-b-bucks*, who has said this while unlocking the brake on the chair, then bringing the chair to a stop in the corridor off the kitchen, beneath a cheap, imitation American Impressionist landscape that hangs in that hallway, just so that he can hug his mom one more time because he hasn't seen her in months, because he is a neglectful son, because her condition is worse, always worse, who has fantasized nonetheless about lashing her chair to a television table on casters so that he can just roll her and the idiot box with its barbiturate programming around the house without having to talk to her because he's been watching this decline for two decades or more and *he's fed up with comforting and self-sacrifice, the very ideas make him sick*, whosoever has settled her in the kitchen by the Formica table and opened the refrigerator looking for some mush that will do the job and on which she will not spend the whole night choking as she sometimes does, so that he then has to use that little medical vacuum-cleaner thing, that dental tool, to remove saliva and food particles from her gullet, tiny degraded hunks of minestrone and baby food, who has tripped briefly over his mother's chair trying to get around it on the way to the chocolate milk in the fridge and jammed his toe, *Shit, shit, shit, sorry, Ma*, who has then changed his mind and fetched therein a six-pack of the finest imported beer purchased earlier at the convenience store in town, and popped open one can for himself and one for his mother, who has then carried the beer to his mother and fitted the end of the straw between her lips, exhorting her to *drink, drink*, while emptying his own fine imported beer in a pair of swallows so that he might move on to the next, who has then hugged his mom (again) feeling, in the flush of processed barley and hops, that his life is withal the best of lives, full of threat and bounty, bad news and good, affluence and penury, the sacred and the profane, the masculine and the feminine, whosoever has, in this instant of sorrow and reverence, *learned the answers* to why roses bloom, why wine-glasses sing, why human lips, when kissed, are so soft, and why parents suffer, *he shall never die.*

His mother's voice, as she hears it now, as she hears herself through the dense matter of her physique, *Hey there, cut it out*, as the beer pours from her mouth and down a dish-towel bib and through the bib to the front of her housedress, soaking through its drab beige design, *Hey!*, her voice is faint and inscrutable, she knows, in the autumn of these neuropathogens, full of mumblings and susurrings, imprecisions, nonsense, phonemic accidents, nonsyntactic vocalizations, unfinished thoughts and sentences; her voice is delivered at an improbably slow velocity, and with evident exertion. She knows. She sends no message but pathos. Her son doesn't understand, for example, that the can of imported beer, mostly emptied upon her now, and trickling along the linoleum floor toward one baseboard, is of no interest to her; her son doesn't understand that she doesn't care for beer any longer, as she never much did, feeling that beer is the beverage of the disadvantaged, not at all the choice *in her day*. The straw falls from her pursed lips, topples out of the can, and cartwheels across her lap, before splashing to rest in the beer pooling by the side of her chair. Her son doesn't understand. He glares at her and carries the empty to a to-be-recycled carton of reinforced cardboard by the back door, and begins again to rummage in the refrigerator. The reason she has summoned him here, having sent home the nurse, Aviva, for the weekend, is among the sentences so far not fully expressed. She is aware of this—as her son, nervously trying to excise a hangnail with his teeth (*Don't hang on the door of the refrigerator, please*, she wants to say), slams the door of same and then lurches out of the kitchen, returning with a bottle of bourbon from the bar in the pantry. Her son tries to anticipate her needs, to preempt her need for words, to eliminate a language based on need, and thus *to eliminate language* (and with it this drama of anguished communication). He reformulates all the conversation into simple yeas or nays. *You d-d-don't want the beer? Are you comfortable? Are you warm enough? D-do you want another light on? Kind of d-dark in here, M-m-mom, isn't it? Do you need to be changed? The nurse t-take you out today?* However, even this simple, binary information system is faulty and replete with misunderstandings. Because her replies, mere probabilities of meaning when you get right down to it, are mostly formulated through *microgesticulations*, a semantics of the faintly conveyed message—the half-closed eyelid, the pressing together of chapped or drooling lips, the head cocked slightly to one side, or the epiglottal choking sound—those communications still permitted by the encrusted linkages of her nerves. This is the foundation of her language now, she is well aware, and therefore it's *the language of mothers and sons*, the language of love between the generations, anyway; all recollections, beseechments, expressions of tenderness, along with her more mundane requests and importunities, must begin with this semantics of gesticulation. Which is to say that speech, for her, is soon going to be a thing of the past. The speech act will follow, into the gloaming, her handwriting, her perfumed thank-you notes, her love letters, her journal entries, her business letters, even her signature, that florid and legally binding evidence of self. Her speech will vanish as these things have vanished. But as her son spoons a few ounces of applesauce into a teacup for her, *My God, applesauce is tedious beyond belief,* the constraint of silence is more than she can bear, suddenly, she just can't relax, and from inside her she tries each muscle, each of her smallest appendages, the knuckle of a toe whose nail had once been painted lavender, a fingertip that once tickled the ivories. In the lockbox where she is located, she focusses all remaining intention on her arm, thinking, feeling, *Dear, there's something I need to tell you. Could you please settle down for just a minute so that I can explain something to you? Could you please stay clearheaded long enough to have a conversation? There is something troubling that I need to ask of you.* She can feel this arm moving, she's sure of it, but when she looks (through trifocal lenses) she can see that it is stationary, this arm is stationary in her lap, white downy fuzz upon alabaster flesh, this flesh wrapped haphazardly, loosely upon the ulna. No muscle to speak of. She tries to reach for him, for her son, but the arm, like the other, sits in her lap, left hand holding the spastic right. The left side of her, where all the remaining movement has been warehoused, can still travel a couple of centimetres to and fro, maybe an inch, but it seems today, when she really needs it, to drowse and idle. When she catches her next head cold or cold sore or is bitten by her next mosquito this mobility will—if the past is any guide—abandon her as it has elsewhere. That's how the disease works. (Here her son sneezes ominously and then looks distractedly around him for a tissue, a strand of mucus yo-yoing from his nose. He staggers to a dish towel, head tilted back, scours his upper lip, and then returns to the applesauce.) Her exertion, though, and the transient paralysis caused by the bath, leave her exhausted, too tired, and she doesn't know if she will be able to get tongue and teeth and breath around the simple magic of a few consonants and vowels. The alphabet is all hairpin turns and pyrotechnical displays. She thinks if there is in her no evidence of any *perceptible* language, who is to blame for that? If perception is required for language, well, then, it's a pretty faulty design. Inside her, language dances on. As does memory. What a rich store of memories she has, outside of what might be heard or seen—as her son fixes himself a drink. What a dance of feelings at the sound of the ice hitting the bottom of the tumbler again. Her son is like his father, as so many sons are, she thinks, and this association leads her astray, this association collides with the present and then darts off parallel, and she follows the past, as she is free to do, until suddenly she comes up short two years ago. *To when they gave her a gift.* Her son and her second husband. It was Christmastime, and they had given her the gift, bought her *a notebook-style computer, Dell Corporation with PMCIA Type II slot and Yamaha YM262 twenty-voice synthesizer and Media Vision pro audio studio*, as her husband had described it, *to be bundled with the popular HandiSpeak software*, mostly portable, mostly wireless, a new prototype, a wireless technology, so that the notebook could sit on top of the tray table on her chair and broadcast a message back to the desktop system (situated on her antique rolltop). What did the facsimile voice sound like? The voice of HandiSpeak? The three of them, she remembers, in the tableau around the Christmas tree in the drafty, poorly lit living room, ceilings too high, tree overdecorated, over-tinselled (by her son), the three of them, pulling the ribbons from *the gift*, well, the men pulling the ribbons from it, herself simply watching, heavy cables and obscure plugs and cords snaking out from under hastily and poorly folded wrapping paper, little seraphic elves dancing on a purple field, pine needles and stray tinsel strands dusting the surface of black and gray plastic casing as they dusted all the surfaces in the living room. They looked at her for approval, and because, back then, two years ago, she still had a little bit of a nod left, *she nodded noncommittally*, and her husband goaded on her son as if he were still a boy and not in his middle thirties, *Go ahead, boot it up*, and he did as he was told, turned on the monitor, shreds of plastic tape still affixed to it like sutures, all the gleaming red operating lamps illumined, and there was the Windows, appearing on the monitor like a reassuring first gasp from an infant, and then the HandiSpeak pointer, with its stylized index finger and rolled-up sleeve. Before them, on the screen (they rolled her closer so she could see), in an ornate computer font—Garamond Antiqua—were the twenty-six letters of the English alphabet, as perfect and simple as atoms must have seemed when Democritus (she thought) imagined them, those simple little squiggles of which arguments were formed, those squiggles that divided houses and united them, that were arranged into the words intoned over baptisms and deaths. Those letters taken from her by her illness. Her son used the mouse apparatus, the ergonomically designed joystick requiring *an absolute minimum of mobility* on the part of its hapless user, and clicked on the alpha of the HandiSpeak alphabet:

> a aback abandon abase abate abbreviate abdicate abdomen abduct aberrant abet abhor ability abject ablaze able abnegate abnormal aboard abode abolish A-bomb abominate abort about above abrasion abscess

abscond absent absolute abstain abstract absurd abuse abusive abysmal
accelerate accent accept acceptance access accessible accident accept acceptance access accessible accident accommodate accost accretion accrue
accumulate accurate accursed accuse ace ache achieve acid acknowledge
acme acorn acoustic acquisition acquit acre acrimony acronym across
act action activate active actor actual actuary acute adagio Adam ada-
mant adapt add addict address adequate adhere adjective adjoin ad-
journ adjunct adjust ad-lib administer admiral admire admit admonish
adolescent adore adorn adornment adrenaline adulate adult adulterate
adultery advance adventure

This forest of "A" words beautiful and strange as he scrolled through
them. Words *were* civilization! And as she gazed on them, on her lost society (though it was obvious that the HandiSpeak's vocabulary had been
culled from one of those inferior college dictionaries), she was, of course,
speechless. Her son eased the joystick through the list, looking for *le mot
juste*, the perfect arrangement of euphony and content, and he settled finally
on one, designating with the pointer the word "adore." Then he selected the
edit menu and designated *Go*.

Adore, the Yamaha YM262 twenty-voice synthesizer's *disembodied
woman's voice* called out from the pile of space junk and wrapping paper on
the Oriental carpet in the living room; the self-assured yet clinical voice
sang out, as though there were a fourth person in the room, an unexpected,
overstaying holiday guest. The voice, as she recollected it, was like nothing so much as the voice of *science*, the voice of technological advancement,
the voice of lasers and digits and particle colliders, of ultra-high-frequency
transmissions. A woman's voice as men would design it. There was a perfume in the room of dying pine. A rich smell. And there was candlelight.
An intimate little fire in the fireplace. And then there was this voice. The
men circled around her trying to gauge her response. They were expectant.
Her son knelt by the computer and clicked on *Return* twice more: *adore,
adore*. The enormity of the machinery was apparent to her at last, what
science could manage, which, in her case, amounted to using fifty pounds
of microchips and motherboards and plastic chassis to enable her to croak
out a few meagre remarks in a prefabricated woman's voice, not her own
voice at all, which had been rich and full, with vigorous laughter, ample
melody—*her voice was gone*. She had been a talker. She had been able to put
the awkward at ease; she had been able to comfort children; she had been
able to sweet-talk truculent shopkeepers. But her voice was gone, was con-
signed now to the netherworld of widowed socks and earrings. She began
to cry, in the living room, and her tears were of the specifically disabled
sort. They came without pounding of fists or oaths, they simply fell, like

summer drizzle, no sound accompanying them, just their erratic progress along her cheeks. *We tried to make sure it was a woman's voice*, her son said, tripping over a coil of patch cords as he made his way to her side, and then her husband said, *Honey, you have to make an effort, you can't just let this happen the way you're doing; we love you, but you have to make an effort. This will help you hang onto your independence, don't you see? Don't you want that? Don't you want to be able to get around in your daily life? I know you do. We know you do. We were thinking about you, honey; we want the best for you, and we got the best, top of the line, the most advanced model. Just give it a try.* And her son said, *If it was up to me, Ma, I would have gotten you an Urdu voice, or a Tibeto-Burman voice, or something, but you can add extra voices, Ma, just the way you can add extra typefaces for your computer. We got an upgrade kit, right there with the software.* But it wasn't the woman's voice—that husky, dental assistant's voice—that put another nail in her pine box. That was just the *perceptible* part of it. The relentless predictability of disabling traumas was *beyond words*, stretched out around her, fore and aft, hemming her in. So why speak at all? *I will not*, she said, *I will not use it. I will not.* And those words *were* properly transmitted. Her husband and her son, they heard her, though they didn't want to. It put a damper on the rest of Christmas Day. When Aviva, the nurse, tried to feed her, at the dining-room table—a morsel of goose speared on the end of a tine—she kept her mouth clamped shut. Like an unruly brat. And since then *the gift* had sat unused, its back-lit, active-matrix screen blinking, waiting for the moment when the affections and recollections of her life would be gobbled by it and converted into the ones and zeroes of a sixteen-bit sound card. Well, as time passed, she did use it occasionally, grudgingly. There was the telephone message. She always wondered why people didn't hang up on it: *Hello, I am temporarily unable to speak with you. My assistant is available, however, if you would care to call again in the early afternoon. Have a wonderful day.* But mostly it was unused, her doppelgänger, though the household current continued to circulate through it. Mostly, her double was silent—that is, until yesterday. Thursday. Which was when Aviva wheeled her up to her desk, and helped her work out the text of her telephone call. She was summoning her boy. Her middle-aged son. Her only child. The son now raising the stainless-steel tablespoon of applesauce toward her mouth, tugging down her chin with one hand, his face close to hers now, the broken blood vessels like a contour map around his nose and under his eyes, his head shorn of all but a faint shadow of his rich chestnut hair, his chin, disgracefully unshaven, with its mix of strawberry-blond and gray hairs, his awkward glasses, from the nineteen-fifties (she guesses), his bloodshot eyes, oh, what has happened to him! How has he begun so suddenly to grow older? When he speaks at last, when he emerges from distraction to see in certain *gesticulations* the fact that an urgency is upon her now, *What is it, Ma? What's wrong? Is there something you want to say?*, when he presses his probably unwashed ear, clotted with earwax, presses it close to her lips, close enough to graze her lips, *then* she begins to feel the reservoir of panic in her, the panic that is like a second inhabitant in this loose garment body, the panic that is never distant, the panic she mostly manages to put aside, but which is now swelling in her like a miraculous pregnancy, *Oh darling*, she says to her son, whispering the words as best she can, a minute elapsing before she can complete the thought, in the stillness of the kitchen, at the beginning of night, with autumn announcing winter, *your mother is in a marvellously big parcel of trouble. I am alone.*

3

The Third Dumpster

& *Gish Jen*

Goodwin Lee and his brother Morehouse had bought it at auction, for nothing. Even the local housing shark had looked down at his list and frowned and pinched or maybe itched his nose, but then waved his hand to clarify: no bid. The house was a dog. However, it had a bedroom on the first floor and was located in the same town as Goodwin and Morehouse.

They were therefore fixing it up for their parents. Goodwin and Morehouse were good with fixer-uppers, after all; they were, in fact, when they were working, contractors. And their parents were *Chinese, end of story*, as Morehouse liked to say. Meaning that though they had been Americans for fifty years and could no longer belay themselves hand over hand up their apartment stair rail to get to their bedroom, they nonetheless could not go into assisted living because of the food. Western food every day? *Cannot eat*, they said.

Goodwin had brought them to a top-notch facility anyway, just to visit. He had pointed out the smooth smooth paths, so wonderful for walking. He had pointed out the wide wide doorways, so open and inviting. And the elevators! Didn't they make you want to go up? He had pointed out the mah-jong. The karaoke. The six-handed pinochle. The senior tai qi. The lobby was full of plants, fake and alive. Always something in bloom! he said, hopefully.

But, distracted as they could be, his parents had frowned undistractedly and replied, *Lamb chops! Salad!* And that was that. His brother, Morehouse, of course, did not entirely comprehend their refusal to eat salad, believing as he did in raw foods. He began every day with a green shake whirled in a blender with an engine like a lawnmower's; the drink looked like a blended lawn, perfect for cows. But never mind. Morehouse accepted, as Goodwin did not quite, that their parents were fundamentally different; their Chineseness was inalienable. Morehouse and Goodwin, on the other hand, would never be *American, end of story*, which was why their parents had never been at a loss for words in their prime. *You are finally learn how to act! You are finally learn how to talk! You are finally learn how to think!* they had said in their kinder moods. Now, though, setting their children straight had at last given way to keeping their medications straight. They also had their sodium levels to think of. One might not think the maintenance of a low-salt diet could be a contribution to inter-generational peace, but, in truth, Goodwin found it made his parents easier to love—more like the diffuse-focus old people of fairy tales, and less like people who above all held steadfast against the irresponsible fanning of their children's self-regard.

The house, however, was a challenge. See these walls? Morehouse had said. And he was right. They were like the walls of a refrigerator box that had been left out in the rain. The bathroom was veined a deep penicillin green; its formerly mauve ceiling was purpurating. Which was why Goodwin was out scouting for dumpsters. Because this was what the recession meant in their neck of the woods: old people moving into purpurating ranch houses unless their unemployed children could do something about it. He did not, of course, like the idea of illicit trash disposal; he would have preferred to do this, as all things, in an above-board manner. But Morehouse had pushed up his sun visor, flashing a Taoist ba gua tattoo, and then held this position as if in a yoga class.

Tell me, he said patiently. Tell me—what choice do we have? Tell me.

The gist of his patience being: Sure it was illegal to use other people's dumpsters, but it was going to save him and Goodwin eight hundred dollars! Eight hundred dollars they didn't have between them, four hundred they didn't have each. It was about dignity for their parents, said Morehouse. It was about doing what they were able to do. It was about doing what sons were bound to do, which was not to pussyfoot around. Morehouse said he would do the actual dumping. Goodwin just had to figure out where other people were having work done, and whether their dumpsters were night-time accessible. As for why Goodwin should do the scouting, that was because Morehouse was good with a sledgehammer and could get the demo started. Goodwin was dangerous with a sledgehammer, especially to himself.

Now he scouted carefully, in his old Corolla wagon, eating Oreos. One dumpster was maybe too close, he thought. Might not its change of fill level be linked with their dumpsterless job right around the corner? Another possibility was farther away. That was a small dumpster, though—too small for the job, really. Someone was being cheap. Also, it was close to a number of houses. People might wake up and hear them.

The third dumpster was a little farther away yet. No houses nearby; that was because it was for the repurposing of a bowling-alley. Who knew what the alley was being repurposed for, but an enormous bowling-pin-shaped sign lay on the ground, leaning horizontally against the cinder-block building. It looked as if the pin had been knocked down for eternity and would never be reset. The dumpster in front of it, in contrast, was fresh and empty, apparently brand new. Bright mailbox-blue, it looked so much more like the Platonic ideal of a dumpster than the real-world item itself that Goodwin found it strangely heartening. Not that he would ever have said so to Morehouse, of course. And, in fact, its pristine state posed a kind of problem, as dumping things into an empty dumpster made noise; the truly ideal dumpster was at least one-quarter full. Goodwin had faith, though, that this one would soon attain that condition. The bowling alley was closed; a construction company had put its sign up by the street. There would be trash. It was true that there were street lights nearby, one of them in working order. That meant Goodwin and Morehouse would not have the cover of darkness. On the other hand, they themselves would be able to see. That was a plus.

At the house, Goodwin found Morehouse out back, receiving black plastic bags full of debris from some workers. The workers lifted them up to him like offerings; he heaved them, in turn, into a truck. Of course, the workers were illegal, as Goodwin well knew. He knew too that Morehouse knew Goodwin to be against the use of illegals, and that Morehouse knew Goodwin knew Morehouse knew that. There was probably no point in even taking him aside. Still, Goodwin took him aside.

Did you really expect me to demo this place all by my friggin' self? asked Morehouse. Anyway, they need the work.

The workers were Guatemalan—open-miened men who nonetheless looked at each other before they said or did anything. Their names were Jose and Ovidio. They shared a water bottle. As Morehouse did not speak Spanish, and the Guatemalans did not speak English, they called him Señor Morehouse and saved their swearing for each other. Goodwin remembered enough from his Vista teaching days to pick up *¡serote!* And *¡hijo de la gran puta!* And *¡que vaina!* Still the demo was apparently going fine. Goodwin watched as they delivered another half-dozen bags of debris to Morehouse.

And that's not even the end of the asbestos, said Morehouse.

Asbestos? cried Goodwin.

You can't be surprised there's asbestos, said Morehouse.

And indeed, Goodwin was not surprised, when he thought about it.

How, though, could Morehouse have asked Jose and Ovidio to remove it? Their lungs! Goodwin objected.

They want to do it, Morehouse shrugged. We paid them extra. They've got it half in the bags already.

But it's illegal!

We have no choice, said Morehouse. And: They have a choice. They don't have to say yes. They can say no.

Are you saying that they are better off than we are? That they have choices where we have none? That is a gross distortion of the situation! argued Goodwin.

Morehouse looked at his watch: time for his seitan burger.

Dumping asbestos is like putting melamine in milk, Goodwin went on. It's like rinsing off IV needles and selling them back to hospitals. It bespeaks the sort of total disregard for public safety that makes one thankful for lawsuits, as Jeannie used to say.

Jeannie was Goodwin's prosecutor ex-wife—a woman of such standards that she'd been through some two or three marriages since theirs. Morehouse smirked with extra zest at the sound of her name.

You seem to think we have no choice, but we absolutely do have a choice, declared Goodwin then. We could, for example, take Mom and Dad in to live with one of us.

For this was the hot truth; it seared him to say it.

Morehouse, though, gave him the look of a man whose wife brought home the bacon now. It was the look of a man who knew what would fly in his house, *end of story*. He lowered his dust mask.

Did you or did you not find a friggin' dumpster? He asked. His mask was not clean, but neither was it caked with dust, like the masks of Jose and Ovidio. What you could see of their faces looked dull and crackled, like ancient earthworks that had started off as mud.

In the end, Goodwin looked the other way as more bags were filled. And though Morehouse had promised to do the dumping, it was Goodwin, finally, who drove the bags to the mailbox-blue dumpster. At least there was, as he predicted, some trash in it now. He did not make much noise as he threw his bags in deep, where they were less likely to be seen by the bowling-alley crew in the morning. The bags were heavy and shifted as if with some low-valence life force. Still, he hurled them as best he could, glad for the working street light but a little paranoid that someone would drive by and see him. No one did. He did think he saw, though, a bit of white smoke rise from the dumpster as he drove away. That was not really possible. The asbestos was in bags, after all; the bags were tied up. He was probably seeing some distortion in the lamplight. And didn't other things send up dust besides asbestos? Sheetrock, for example. Sheetrock sent up dust. Still, he thought he saw asbestos rising up on that dump, and on another dump he made before switching to yet another dumpster he had found, behind a Masonic temple. He didn't think there was asbestos in any of the new bags of trash, but who knew? He didn't ask, and Morehouse didn't say.

In a further effort to save money, Goodwin and Morehouse roughed out the walls themselves; and though they didn't have an electrician's license, they took care of the wiring too. They even set a new used cast-iron tub, or tried to. In fact, they got it three inches too high and had to turn once again to Jose and Ovidio for help getting the thing back out. Of course, Jose and Ovidio shook their heads and laughed when they saw what had happened. *¡Que jodida!* they said. Then they spent an entire day grimacing and straining, their faces almost as purple as the ceiling. When the tub finally rested back on a pallet in the hall, Ovidio stared at it a long moment. *¡Tu madre!* he muttered, to which Jose swore back *¡La tuya!*, his arms jerking up and down, his neck twitching with anger. He pulled up his pants, maybe because they were too big; Goodwin made a mental note to bring him a belt, though what Jose and Ovidio probably needed was more food. Would Goodwin have been right to insist, as he wanted to, on finishing the job without them? After they'd already helped with the dirtiest and most grueling parts? He decided to let Morehouse have his way, and had to admit that Jose, at least, looked happy to have the work. Goodwin gave him a belt, which he seemed to appreciate; he slipped both men an extra twenty too. Take it, Goodwin told them. *Por favor.*

Was this why the work went quickly and well? And yet, still, Morehouse and Goodwin kept their parents from the site for as long as possible, knowing that something about the project was bound to spark their disapproval. *House cost nothing, but look how much you spend on renovation,* their mother might say. Or, *How come even you have no job, you hire other people to work?* Morehouse, naturally, was well stocked with rebuttals, starting with, *Don't worry, we barely pay these workers anything.* What difference these could make, though, was unclear.

Finally, though, it couldn't be helped; their parents came for a visit. They looked around stupefied. The house was not much bigger than their apartment, but it was big enough to make them seem smaller; and all new as it was, it made them look older.

Very nice, said their mother finally. She clutched her leather-trim pocketbook as if to ward off attackers; she showed real excitement about the window in the bathroom and the heating ducts. *No radiators!* she exclaimed. Their father looked as much at Jose and Ovidio as the house. *Spanish guys*, he said. Jose and Ovidio laughed and kept working. Goodwin tried to explain what they were doing. What the house used to look like. What it was going to look like. And how much they, his parents, were going to like it. It was like trying to sell them on the assisted-living place. Everything on one floor! Close to their sons! Right in the same town! His pitch was so good that Morehouse stopped and listened—suddenly touched himself, it seemed, by what they had wrought. He beamed as if to say, Behold what we've done for you! He leaned toward their shuffling father, as if expecting to hear, What great sons you boys are!

Instead their father tripped over a toolbox and fell as if hit by a sledgehammer. Dad? Dad? He was conscious but open-mouthed and breathing hard; there was some blood, but only, Goodwin was relieved to see, a little. *I fine*, he insisted, flapping a shaking hand in the vicinity of his hip. Your hip? asked Goodwin. Their father nodded a little, grimacing—his brown age spots growing prominent as his real self, it seemed, paled. Don't move, it's OK, said Goodwin. It's OK. And, to Morehouse: Do you have an ice pack in your lunch box?

Morehouse called an ambulance. People said the ambulance service was quick around here, or could be; that was reassuring. As he and his family waited, though, Goodwin stared at his father lying on the floor, and was shocked at how like a house that could not be fixed up he seemed. He started into the air with his milky eyes as if he did not want any of them to be there and, oddly, covered his mouth with his still-trembling hand. It was a thing he did now at funny times, as if he knew how yellow his teeth were; or maybe it was something else. Goodwin's father had always been a mystery. Now he was more manifestly obscured than ever. The few things he said were like ever darkening peepholes into fathomless depths. *You don't know what old is*, he said sometimes. *Everything take long time. Long, long time.* And once, simply: *No fun.*

His more demonstrative mother cried the whole way to the hospital, saying that his father fell because he didn't want to move into this house, and that she didn't either. It was her way of making herself clear. She didn't care whether or not it was the sort of house a person could live in by herself one day, she said. Chinese people, she said, did not live by themselves.

They were passing the turn-off for Goodwin's house when she said that. Goodwin was glad they were in an ambulance. He smiled reassuringly at his father though his eyes were closed tight; he had an oxygen mask on.

Right now we need to focus on Dad, Goodwin said.

His mother would not take her pocketbook off her lap.

Morehouse, following them in his car so that they would have a car at the hospital, called Goodwin on his cellphone.

If they ask whether dad needs a translator tell them to fuck off, he said.

Does he need a translator? asked the admitting nurse.

He's lived here for fifty years, answered Goodwin politely.

The nurse was at least a grown-up. The doctor looked like a paper boy.

Does he need a translator? he asked.

Fuck off, said Morehouse, walking in.

How Goodwin wished he had said that! And how much he wished he had ended up like Morehouse instead of like Morehouse inside out. For maybe if he had, he would not have sat in the waiting room later, endlessly hearing what his mother wanted him to say—*You guys can come live with me*—much less what she would say if he said it: *You are finally learn how to take care of people. Who knows, maybe next time your wife get divorced, she come back, marry you again.*

Instead his mother was probably going to say, *You know why your wife dump you? She is completely American, that's why. Even she marry you gain, she just dump you again. You wait and see.*

Fuck off, he would want to say then, like Morehouse. Fuck off!

But, of course, not even Morehouse would say that to their mother any more. Now, in deference to her advanced and ever-advancing age, even Morehouse would probably nod and agree. Their mother would say, *That's what American people are. Dump people like garbage. That's what they are.*

And Morehouse would answer, *That's what they are, all right, the fuckers.*

Nodding and nodding, even as he went on building.

4

Water

❧ *Li-Young Lee*

The sound of 36 pines side by side surrounding
the yard and swaying all night like individual
   hymns is the sound
of water, which is the oldest sound,
the first sound we forgot.

At the ocean
my brother stands in water
to his knees, his chest bare, hard, his arms
thick and muscular. He is no swimmer.
In water
my sister is no longer
lonely. Her right leg is crooked and smaller
than her left, but she swims straight.
Her whole body is a glimmering fish.

Water is my father's life-sign.
Son of water who'll die by water,
the element which rules his life shall take it.
After being told so by a wise man in Shantung,
after almost drowning twice,
he avoided water. But the sign of water
is a flowing sign, going where its children go.

Water has invaded my father's
heart, swollen, heavy,
twice as large. Bloated

liver. Bloated legs.
The feet have become balloons.
A respirator mask makes him look
like a diver. When I lay my face
against his—the sound of water
returning.

The sound of washing
is the sound of sighing,
is the only sound
as I wash my father's feet—those lonely twins
who have forgotten one another
one by one in warm water
I tested with my wrist.
In soapy water
they're two dumb fish
whose eyes close in a filmy dream.

I dry, then powder them
with talc rising in clouds
like dust lifting
behind jeeps, a truck where he sat
bleeding through his socks.
1949, he's 30 years old,
his toenails pulled out,

his toes beaten a beautiful
violet that reminds him
Of Hunan, barely morning
in the yard, and where
he walked, the grass springing back
damp and green.

The sound of rain
outlives us. I listen,
someone is whispering.
Tonight, it's water
the curtains resemble, water
drumming on the steel cellar door, water
we crossed to come to America,
water I'll cross to go back,
water which will kill my father.
The sac of water we live in.

5

Lucky

ℰ *Tony Hoagland*

If you are lucky in this life,
you will get to help your enemy
the way I got to help my mother
when she was weakened past the point of saying no.

Into the big enamel tub
half-filled with water
which I had made just right,
I lowered the childish skeleton
she had become.

Her eyelids fluttered as I soaped and rinsed
her belly and her chest,
the sorry ruin of her flanks
and the frayed gray cloud
between her legs.

Some nights, sitting by her bed
book open in my lap
while I listened to the air
move thickly in and out of her dark lungs,
my mind filled up with praise
as lush as music,

amazed at the symmetry and luck
that would offer me the chance to pay

my heavy debt of punishment and love
with love and punishment.

And once I held her dripping wet
in the uncomfortable air
between the wheelchair and the tub,
until she begged me like a child

to stop,
an act of cruelty which we both understood
was the ancient irresistible rejoicing
of power over weakness.

If you are lucky in this life,
you will get to raise the spoon
of pristine, frosty ice cream
to the trusting creature mouth
of your old enemy

because the tastebuds at least are not broken
because there is a bond between you
and sweet is sweet in any language.

6

Fathers and Sons

❧ David Mason

Some things, they say,
one should not write about. I tried
to help my father comprehend
the toilet, how one needs
to undo one's belt, to slide
one's trousers down and sit,
but he stubbornly stood
and would not bend his knees.
I tried again
to bend him toward the seat,

and then I laughed
at the absurdity. Fathers and sons.
How he had wiped my bottom
half a century ago, and how
I would repay the favor
if he would only sit.

Don't you—
he gripped me, trembling, searching for my eyes.
Don't you—but the word
was lost to him. Somewhere
a man of dignity would not be laughed at.
He could not see
it was the crazy dance
that made me laugh,
trying to make him sit
when he wanted to stand.

7

Yesterday

❧ *W. S. Merwin*

My friend says I was not a good son
you understand
I say yes I understand

he says I did not go
to see my parents very often you know
and I say yes I know

even when I was living in the same city he says
maybe I would go there once
a month or maybe even less
I say oh yes

he says the last time I went to see my father
I say the last time I saw my father

he says the last time I saw my father
he was asking me about my life
how I was making out and he
went into the next room
to get something to give me

oh I say
feeling again the cold
of my father's hand the last time
he says and my father turned
in the doorway and saw me
look at my wristwatch and he

---

said you know I would like you to stay
and talk with me

oh yes I say

but if you are busy he said
I don't want you to feel that you
have to
just because I'm here

I say nothing

he says my father
said maybe
you have important work you are doing
or maybe you should be seeing
somebody I don't want to keep you

I look out the window
my friend is older than I am
he says and I told my father it was so
and I got up and left him then
you know

though there was nowhere I had to go
and nothing I had to do

8

Ode to Meaning

❦ Robert Pinsky

Dire one and desired one,
Savior, sentencer—

In an old allegory you would carry
A chained alphabet of tokens:

Ankh Badge Cross.
Dragon,
Engraved figure guarding a hallowed intaglio,
Jasper kinema of legendary Mind,
Naked omphalos pierced
By quills of rhyme or sense, torah-like: unborn
Vein of will, xenophile
Yearning out of Zero.

Untrusting I court you. Wavering
I seek your face, I read
That Crusoe's knife
Reeked of you, that to defile you
The soldier makes the rabbi spit on the torah.
"I'll drown my book" says Shakespeare.

Drowned walker, revenant.
After my mother fell on her head, she became
More than ever your sworn enemy. She spoke
Sometimes like a poet or critic of forty years later.
Or she spoke of the world as Thersites spoke of the heroes,

"I think they have swallowed one another. I
Would laugh at that miracle."

You also in the laughter, warrior angel:
Your helmet the zodiac, rocket-plumed
Your spear the beggar's finger pointing to the mouth
Your heel planted on the serpent Formulation
Your face a vapor, the wreath of
    cigarette smoke crowning
Bogart as he winces through it.

Torsion, a cleavage
Stirring even in the arctic ice,
Even at the dark ocean floor, even
In the cellular flesh of a stone.

Gas. Gossamer. My poker friends
Question your presence
In a poem by me, passing the magazine
One to another.

Not the stone and not the words, you
Like a veil over Arthur's headstone,
The passage from Proverbs he chose
While he was too ill to teach
And still well enough to read, *I was*
Beside the master craftsman
Delighting him day after day, ever
At play in his presence—you

A soothing veil of distraction playing over
Dying Arthur playing in the hospital,
Thumbing the Bible, fuzzy from medication,
Ever courting your presence,
And you the prognosis,
You in the cough.

Gesturer, when is your spur, your cloud?
You in the airport rituals of greeting and parting.
Indicter, who is your claimant?
Bell at the gate. Spiderweb iron bridge.
Cloak, video, aroma, rue, what is your
Elected silence, where was your seed?

What is Imagination
But your lost child born to give birth to you?

Dire one. Desired one.
Savior, sentencer—

Absence,
Or presence ever at play:
Let those scorn you who never
Starved in your dearth. If I
Dare to disparage
Your harp of shadows I taste
Wormwood and motor oil, I pour
Ashes on my head. You are the wound. You
Be the medicine.

9

Buckdancer's Choice

❧ *James Dickey*

So I would hear out those lungs,
The air split into nine levels,
Some gift of tongues of the whistler

In the invalid's bed: my mother,
Warbling all day to herself
The thousand variations of one song;

It is called Buckdancer's Choice.
For years, they have all been dying
Out, the classic buck-and-wing men

Of traveling minstrel shows;
With them also an old woman
Was dying of breathless angina,

Yet still found breath enough
To whistle up in my head
A sight like a one-man band,

Freed black, with cymbals at heel,
An ex-slave who thrivingly danced
To the ring of his own clashing light

Through the thousand variations of one song
All day to my mother's prone music,
The invalid's warbler's note,

While I crept close to the wall
Sock-footed, to hear the sounds alter,
Her tongue like a mockingbird's break

Through stratum after stratum of a tone
Proclaiming what choices there are
For the last dancers of their kind,

For ill women and for all slaves
Of death, and children enchanted at walls
With a brass-beating glow underfoot,

Not dancing but nearly risen
Through barnlike, theatrelike houses
On the wings of the buck and wing.

10

Where the Groceries Went

❧ *Raymond Carver*

When his mother called for the second time
that day, she said:
"I don't have any strength left. I want
to lay down all the time."

"Did you take your iron?" he wanted to know.
He sincerely wanted to know. Praying daily,
hopelessly, that iron might make a difference.
"Yes, but it just makes me hungry. And I don't
have anything to eat."

He pointed out to her they'd shopped
for hours that morning. Brought home
eighty dollars' worth of food to stack
in her cupboards and the fridge.
"There's nothing to eat in this goddamn house
but baloney and cheese," she said.
Her voice shook with anger. "Nothing!"
"And how's your cat? How's Kitty doing?"
His own voice shook. He needed
to get off this subject of food; it never
brought them anything but grief.

"Kitty," his mother said. "Here, Kitty.
Kitty, Kitty. She won't answer me, honey.
I don't know this for sure, but I think
she jumped into the washing machine
when I was about to do a load. And before I forget,
that machine's making
a banging noise. I think there's something
the matter with it. Kitty! She won't
answer me. Honey, I'm afraid.
I'm afraid of everything. Help me please.
Then you can go back to whatever it was
you were doing. Whatever
it was that was so important
I had to take the trouble
to bring you into this world."

PART II

Husbands and Wives

Part of the traditional marriage ceremony is the vow each partner makes to take care of each other "in sickness and in health." It is appropriate that "in sickness" comes first, because illness or disability challenges marriages in profound ways. Illness upsets the existing emotional, financial, and power balance that partners create, perhaps unconsciously. The selections in this section illustrate some of the ways different spouses respond to these changing roles and relationships.

In "Mrs. Cassidy's Last Year" by Mary Gordon, Mr. Cassidy tests the limits of his vow, made when he and his wife were in their thirties, to let her die in her own bed. But now she is demented, foul-mouthed, and violent. His Catholic faith will not let him go back on his promise but "he had sinned against charity. He wanted his wife dead." His son and his son's wife want him to place Rose in a nursing home, but he resists until the inevitable crisis.

Ethan Canin's story "We are Nighttime Travelers" is another examination of a couple's adjustment to dementia. The husband, after forty-six years of marriage, says, "This is a love story," but he admits, "Let us say that for the last year I haven't loved her; let us say this for the last ten, even." His wife Francine believes that someone is lurking outside the house. As the husband stands watch for the nonexistent prowler, he re-examines his own life and their marriage. His own illness—a serious case of diabetes—is a recurring theme in the story.

Two sets of poems follow these stories. Donald Hall's poem "The Ship Pounding" likens a hospital where his wife lays ill to a ship whose "passengers on this voyage / wore masks or cannulae / or dangled devices that dripped / chemicals into their wrists." In a companion poem, his wife, the late poet Jane Kenyon, describes life as "The Sick Wife." The pulsing rhythm of Hall's poem is juxtaposed with Kenyon's slow, sad lines about ordinary things she can no longer do.

"Alzheimer's: The Wife" and "Alzheimer's: The Husband," by C. K. Williams portray the dual impact of this disease on the wife with dementia and the husband, who is now faced with spending "his long anticipated retirement learning to cook, / clean house, dress her, even to apply her makeup . . . / . . . the next necessity he saw himself as being called to."

Alice Munro's story, "The Bear Came Over the Mountain," is probably the most familiar story in this book; it has been seen by many people in its film version *Away From Her*. The title of the short story is ambiguous. Does it refer to the children's song, "The Bear Went Over the Mountain," about a bear who wanted "to see what he could see"? Munro has not explained. Perhaps it is simply a variation of the familiar adage that "what goes around comes around." Grant, a retired college professor, has been married to Fiona for years. Fiona is losing her memory and moves to assisted living, where she develops a close friendship with Aubrey. But Aubrey's wife takes him home because she cannot afford to keep him there. Grant's many infidelities now come back to haunt him, and he seeks a familiar resolution to his need to keep Fiona happy.

Another story, "Thoreau's Laundry" by Ann Harleman, also deals with infidelity and illness but with younger protagonists. Celia, the narrator, is a "maxillofacial prosthetist," a technician who makes artificial parts for patients with facial trauma. Her husband Simon has multiple sclerosis and needs constant care. While Celia tends devotedly to Simon, she matter-of-factly describes her lovers, the latest of whom is Max. This story is unusual in that the caregiver also has a working life, which figures prominently in the story. It is also a caregiving story within a caregiving story, as Celia works with a young client and his suspicious mother to gain their trust in her ability to create a prosthetic ear.

Rachel Hadas's poem "The Yawn" introduces another person in the caregiving dyad—her son, who makes her laugh when he yawns like his father. The "orphaned piano"—which her husband played—yawns too in echo. "Mrs. Dumpty," by Chana Bloch, takes the familiar nursery rhyme character and turns Humpty into a broken man and herself into his restorer. A second poem by Bloch, "Visiting Hours Are Over," conveys the common feeling of release after leaving the hospital.

In perhaps the most graphic description of illness in the book, yet also one of the most loving accounts, Anne Brashler's story "He Read to Her" describes a wife's dismay, even disgust, at her body altered by a colostomy. Yet her husband comforts her by demonstrating the theme of this collection—the power of literature to overcome sorrow.

11

Mrs. Cassidy's Last Year

 Mary Gordon

Mr. Cassidy knew he couldn't go to Communion. He had sinned against charity. He had wanted his wife dead.

The intention had been his, and the desire. She would not go back to bed. She had lifted the table that held her breakfast (it was unfair, it was unfair to all of them, that the old woman should be so strong and so immobile). She had lifted the table above her head and sent it crashing to the floor in front of him.

"Rose," he had said, bending, wondering how he would get scrambled egg, coffee, cranberry juice (which she had said she liked, the color of it) out of the garden pattern on the carpet. That was the sort of thing she knew but would not tell him now. She would laugh, wicked and bland faced as an egg, when he did the wrong thing. But never say what was right, although she knew it, and her tongue was not dead for curses, for reports of crimes.

"Shithawk," she would shout at him from her bedroom. "Bastard son of a whore." Or more mildly, "Pimp," or "Fathead fart."

Old words, curses heard from soldiers on the boat or somebody's street children. Never spoken by her until now. Punishing him, though he had kept his promise.

He was trying to pick up the scrambled eggs with a paper napkin. The napkin broke, then shredded when he tried to squeeze the egg into what was left of it. He was on his knees on the carpet, scraping egg, white shreds of paper, purple fuzz from the trees in the carpet.

"Shitscraper," she laughed at him on his knees.

And then he wished in his heart most purely for the woman to be dead.

The doorbell rang. His son and his son's wife. Shame that they should see him so, kneeling, bearing curses, cursing in his heart.

"Pa," said Toni, kneeling next to him. "You see what we mean."

"She's too much for you," said Mr. Cassidy's son Tom. Self-made man, thought Mr. Cassidy. Good time Charlie. Every joke a punchline like a whip.

No one would say his wife was too much for him.

"Swear," she had said, lying next to him in bed when they were each no more than thirty. Her eyes were wild then. What had made her think of it? No sickness near them, and fearful age some continent like Africa, with no one they knew well. What had put the thought to her, and the wildness, so that her nails bit into his palm, as if she knew small pain would preserve his memory.

"Swear you will let me die in my own bed. Swear you won't let them take me away."

He swore, her nails making dents in his palms, a dull shallow pain, not sharp, blue-green or purplish.

He had sworn.

On his knees now beside his daughter-in-law, his son.

"She is not too much for me. She is my wife."

"Leave him then, Toni," said Tom. "Let him do it himself if it's so god-damn easy. Serve him right. Let him learn the hard way. He couldn't do it if he didn't have us, the slobs around the corner."

Years of hatred now come out, punishing for not being loved best, of the family's children not most prized. Nothing is forgiven, thought the old man, rising to his feet, his hand on his daughter-in-law's squarish shoulder.

He knelt before the altar of God. The young priest, bright-haired, faced them, arms open, a good little son.

No sons priests. He thought how he was old enough now to have a priest a grandson. This boy before him, vested and ordained, could have been one of the ones who followed behind holding tools. When there was time. He thought of Tom looking down at his father who knelt trying to pick up food. Tom for whom there had been no time. Families were this: the bulk, the knot of memory, wounds remembered not only because they had set on the soft, the pliable wax of childhood, motherhood, fatherhood, closeness to death. Wounds most deeply set and best remembered because families are days, the sameness of days and words, hammer blows, smothering, breath grabbed, memory on the soft skull, in the lungs, not once only but again and again the same. The words and the starvation.

Tom would not forget, would not forgive him. Children thought themselves the only wounded.

Should we let ourselves in for it, year after year, he asked in prayer, believing God did not hear him.

Tom would not forgive him for being the man he was. A man who paid debts, kept promises. Mr. Cassidy knelt up straighter, proud of himself before God.

Because of the way he had to be. He knelt back again, not proud. As much sense to be proud of the color of his hair. As much choice.

It was his wife who was the proud one. As if she thought it could have been some other way. The house, the children. He knew, being who they were they must have a house like that, children like that. Being who they were to the world. Having their faces.

As if she thought with some wrong turning these things might have been wasted. Herself a slattern, him drunk, them living in a tin shack, children dead or missing.

One was dead. John, the favorite, lost somewhere in a plane. The war dead. There was his name on the plaque near the altar. With the other town boys. And she had never forgiven him. For what he did not know. For helping bring that child into the world? Better, she said, to have borne none than the pain of losing this one, the most beautiful, the bravest. She turned from him then, letting some shelf drop, like a merchant at the hour of closing. And Tom had not forgotten the grief at his brother's death, knowing he could not have closed his mother's heart like that.

Mr. Cassidy saw they were all so unhappy, hated each other so because they thought things could be different. As he had thought of his wife. He had imagined she could be different if she wanted to. Which had angered him. Which was not, was almost never, the truth about things.

Things were as they were going to be, he thought, watching the boy-faced priest giving out Communion. Who were the others not receiving? Teenagers, pimpled, believing themselves in sin. He wanted to tell them they were not. He was sure they were not. Mothers with babies. Not going to Communion because they took the pill, it must be. He thought they should not stay away, although he thought they should not do what they had been told not to. He knew that the others in their seats were there for the heat of their bodies. While he sat back for the coldness of his heart, a heart that had wished his wife dead. He had wished the one dead he had promised he would love forever.

The boy priest blessed the congregation. Including Mr. Cassidy himself.

"Pa," said Tom, walking beside his father, opening the car door for him. "You see what we mean about her?"

"It was my fault. I forgot."

"Forgot what?" said Tom, emptying his car ashtray onto the church parking lot. Not my son, thought Mr. Cassidy, turning his head.

"How she is," said Mr. Cassidy. "I lost my temper."

"Pa, you're not God," said Tom. His hands were on the steering wheel, angry. His mother's.

"Okay," said Toni. "But look, Pa, you've been a saint to her. But she's not the woman she was. Not the woman we knew."

"She's the woman I married."

"Not anymore," said Toni, wife of her husband.

If not, then who? People were the same. They kept their bodies. They did not become someone else. Rose was the woman he had married, a green girl, high-colored, with beautifully cut nostrils, hair that fell down always, hair she pinned up swiftly, with anger. She had been a housemaid and he a chauffeur. He had taken her to the ocean. They wore straw hats. They were not different people now. She was the girl he had seen first, the woman he had married, the mother of his children, the woman he had promised: Don't let them take me. Let me die in my own bed.

"Supposing it was yourself and Tom, then, Toni," said Mr. Cassidy, remembering himself a gentleman. "What would you want him to do? Would you want him to break his promise?"

"I hope I'd never make him promise anything like that," said Toni.

"But if you did?"

"I don't believe in those kinds of promises."

"My father thinks he's God. You have to understand. There's no two ways about anything."

For what was his son now refusing to forgive him? He was silent now, sitting in the back of the car. He looked at the top of his daughter-in-law's head, blond now, like some kind of circus candy. She had never been blond. Why did they do it? Try to be what they were not born to. Rose did not.

"What I wish you'd get through your head, Pa, is that it's me and Toni carrying the load. I suppose you forget where all the suppers come from?"

"I don't forget."

"Why don't you think of Toni for once?"

"I think of her, Tom, and you too. I know what you do. I'm very grateful. Mom is grateful, too, or she would be."

But first I think of my wife to whom I made vows. And whom I promised.

"The doctor thinks you're nuts, you know that, don't you?" said Tom. "Rafferty thinks you're nuts to try and keep her. He thinks we're nuts to go along with you. He says he washes his hands of the whole bunch of us."

The doctor washes his hands, thought Mr. Cassidy, seeing Leo Rafferty, hale as a dog, at his office sink.

The important thing was not to forget she was the woman he had married.

So he could leave the house, so he could leave her alone, he strapped her into the bed. Her curses were worst when he released her. She had grown a beard this last year, like a goat.

Like a man?

No.

He remembered her as she was when she was first his wife. A white nightgown, then as now. So she was the same. He'd been told it smelled different a virgin's first time. And never that way again. Some blood. Not much. As if she hadn't minded.

He sat her in the chair in front of the television. They had Mass now on television for sick people, people like her. She pushed the button on the little box that could change channels from across the room. One of their grandsons was a TV repairman. He had done it for them when she got sick. She pushed the button to a station that showed cartoons. Mice in capes, cats outraged. Some stories now with colored children. He boiled an egg for her lunch.

She sat chewing, looking at the television. What was that look in her eyes now? Why did he want to call it wickedness? Because it was blank and hateful. Because there was no light. Eyes should have light. There should be something behind them. That was dangerous, nothing behind her eyes but hate. Sullen like a bull kept from a cow. Sex mad. Why did that look make him think of sex? Sometimes he was afraid she wanted it.

He did not know what he would do.

She slept. He slept in the chair across from her.

The clock went off for her medicine. He got up from the chair, gauging the weather. Sometimes the sky was green this time of year. It was warm when it should not be. He didn't like that. The mix-up made him shaky. It made him say to himself, "Now I am old."

He brought her the medicine. Three pills, red and grey, red and yellow, dark pink. Two just to keep her quiet. Sometimes she sucked them and spat them out when they melted and she got the bad taste. She thought they were candy. It was their fault for making them those colors. But it was something else he had to think about. He had to make sure she swallowed them right away.

Today she was not going to swallow. He could see that by the way her eyes looked at the television. The way she set her mouth so he could see what she had done with the pills, kept them in a pocket in her cheek, as if for storage.

"Rose," he said, stepping between her and the television, breaking her gaze. "You've got to swallow the pills. They cost money."

She tried to look over his shoulder. On the screen an ostrich, dressed in colored stockings, danced down the road. He could see she was not listening to him. And he tried to remember what the young priest had said when he came to bring Communion, what his daughter June had said. Be patient with her. Humor her. She can't help what she does. She's not the woman she once was.

She is the same.

"Hey, my Rose, won't you just swallow the pills for me. Like my girl."

She pushed him out of the way. So she could go on watching the television. He knelt down next to her.

"Come on, girleen. It's the pills make you better."

She gazed over the top of his head. He stood up, remembering what was done to animals.

He stroked her throat as he had stroked the throats of dogs and horses, a boy on a farm. He stroked the old woman's loose, papery throat, and said, "Swallow, then, just swallow."

She looked over his shoulder at the television. She kept the pills in a corner of her mouth.

It was making him angry. He put one finger above her lip under her nose and one below her chin, so that she would not be able to open her mouth. She breathed through her nose like a patient animal. She went on looking at the television. She did not swallow.

"You swallow them, Rose, this instant," he said, clamping her mouth shut. "They cost money. The doctor says you must. You're throwing good money down the drain."

Now she was watching a lion and polar bear dancing. There were pianos in their cages.

He knew he must move away or his anger would make him do something. He had promised he would not be angry. He would remember who she was.

He went into the kitchen with a new idea. He would give her something sweet that would make her want to swallow. There was ice cream in the refrigerator. Strawberry that she liked. He removed each strawberry and placed it in the sink so she would not chew and then get the taste of the medicine. And then spit it out, leaving him, leaving them both no better than when they began.

He brought the dish of ice cream to her in the living room. She was sitting staring at the television with her mouth open. Perhaps she had opened her mouth to laugh? At what? At what was this grown woman laughing? A zebra was playing a xylophone while his zebra wife hung striped pajamas on a line.

In opening her mouth, she had let the pills fall together onto her lap. He saw the three of them, wet, stuck together, at the center of her lap. He thought he would take the pills and simply hide them in the ice cream. He bent to fish them from the valley of her lap.

And then she screamed at him. And then she stood up.

He was astonished at her power. She had not stood by herself for seven months. She put one arm in front of her breasts and raised the other against him, knocking him heavily to the floor.

"No," she shouted, her voice younger, stronger, the voice of a well young man. "Don't think you can have it now. That's what you're after. That's what you're always after. You want to get into it. I'm not one of your whores. You always thought it was such a great prize. I wish you'd have it cut off. I'd like to cut it off."

And she walked out of the house. He could see her wandering up and down the street in the darkness.

He dragged himself over to the chair and propped himself against it so he could watch her through the window. But he knew he could not move any farther. His leg was light and foolish underneath him, and burning with pain. He could not move any more, not even to the telephone that was half a yard away from him. He could see her body, visible through her nightgown, as she walked the street in front of the house.

He wondered if he should call out or be silent. He did not know how far she would walk. He could imagine her walking until the land stopped, and then into the water. He could not stop her. He would not raise his voice.

There was that pain in his leg that absorbed him strangely, as if it were the pain of someone else. He knew the leg was broken. "I have broken my leg," he kept saying to himself, trying to connect the words and the burning.

But then he remembered what it meant. He would not be able to walk. He would not be able to take care of her.

"Rose," he shouted, trying to move toward the window.

And then, knowing he could not move and she could not hear him, "Help."

He could see the green numbers on the clock, alive as cat's eyes. He could see his wife walking in the middle of the street. At least she was not walking far. But no one was coming to help her.

He would have to call for help. And he knew what it meant: they would take her away somewhere. No one would take care of her in the house if he did not. And he could not move.

No one could hear him shouting. No one but he could see his wife, wandering up and down the street in her nightgown.

They would take her away. He could see it; he could hear the noises.

Policemen in blue, car radios reporting other disasters, young boys writing his words down in notebooks. And doctors, white coats, white shoes, wheeling her out. Her strapped. She would curse him. She would curse him rightly for having broken his promise. And the young men would wheel her out. Almost everyone was younger than he now. And he could hear how she would be as they wheeled her past him, rightly cursing.

Now he could see her weaving in the middle of the street. He heard a car slam on its brakes to avoid her. He thought someone would have to stop then. But he heard the car go on down to the corner.

No one could hear him shouting in the living room. The windows were shut; it was late October. There was a high bulk of grey cloud, showing islands of fierce, acidic blue. He would have to do something to get someone's attention before the sky became utterly dark and the drivers could not see her wandering before their cars. He could see her wandering; he could see the set of her angry back. She was wearing only her nightgown. He would have to get someone to bring her in before she died of cold.

The only objects he could reach were the figurines that covered the low table beside him. He picked one up: a bust of Robert Kennedy. He threw it through the window. The breaking glass made a violent, disgraceful noise. It was the sound of disaster he wanted. It must bring help.

He lay still for ten minutes, waiting, looking at the clock. He could see her walking, cursing. She could not hear him. He was afraid no one could hear him. He picked up another figurine, a bicentennial eagle and threw it through the window next to the one he had just broken. Then he picked up another and threw it through the window next to that. He went on: six windows. He went on until he had broken every window in the front of the house.

He had ruined his house. The one surprising thing of his long lifetime. The broken glass winked like green jewels, hard sea creatures, on the purple carpet. He looked at what he had destroyed. He would never have done it; it was something he would never have done. But he would not have believed he was a man who could not keep his promise.

In the dark he lay and prayed that someone would come and get her. That was the only thing now to pray for; the one thing he had asked God to keep back. A car stopped in front of the house. He heard his son's voice speaking to his mother. He could see the two of them; Tom had his arm around her. She was walking into the house now as if she had always meant to.

Mr. Cassidy lay back for the last moment of darkness. Soon the room would be full.

His son turned on the light.

12

We Are Nighttime Travelers

❧ *Ethan Canin*

Where are we going? Where, I might write, is this path leading us? Francine is asleep and I am standing downstairs in the kitchen with the door closed and the light on and a stack of mostly blank paper on the counter in front of me. My dentures are in a glass by the sink. I clean them with a tablet that bubbles in the water, and although they were clean already I just cleaned them again because the bubbles are agreeable and I thought their effervescence might excite me to action. By action, I mean I thought they might excite me to write. But words fail me.

This is a love story. However, its roots are tangled and involve a good bit of my life, and when I recall my life my mood turns sour and I am reminded that no man makes truly proper use of his time. We are blind and small-minded. We are dumb as snails and as frightened, full of vanity and misinformed about the importance of things. I'm an average man, without great deeds except maybe one, and that has been to love my wife.

I have been more or less faithful to Francine since I married her. There has been one transgression—leaning up against a closet wall with a red-haired purchasing agent at a sales meeting once in Minneapolis twenty years ago; but she was buying auto upholstery and I was selling it and in the eyes of judgment this may bear a key weight. Since then, though, I have ambled on this narrow path of life bound to one woman. This is a triumph and a regret. In our current state of affairs it is a regret because in life a man is either on the uphill or on the downhill, and if he isn't procreating he is on the downhill. It is a steep downhill indeed. These days I am tumbling, falling headlong among the scrub oaks and boulders, tearing my knees and abrading all the bony parts of the body. I have given myself to gravity.

Francine and I are married now forty-six years, and I would be a bamboozler to say that I have loved her for any more than half of these. Let us say that for the last year I haven't; let us say this for the last ten, even. Time has made torments of our small differences and tolerance of our passions.

This is our state of affairs. Now I stand by myself in our kitchen in the middle of the night; now I lead a secret life. We wake at different hours now, sleep in different corners of the bed. We like different foods and different music, keep our clothing in different drawers, and if it can be said that either of us has aspirations, I believe that they are to a different bliss. Also, she is healthy and I am ill. And as for conversation—that feast of reason, that flow of the soul—our house is silent as the bone yard.

Last week we did talk. "Frank," she said one evening at the table, "there is something I must tell you."

The New York game was on the radio, snow was falling outside, and the pot of tea she had brewed was steaming on the table between us. Her medicine and my medicine were in little paper cups at our places.

"Frank," she said, jiggling her cup, "what I must tell you is that someone was around the house last night."

I tilted my pills onto my hand. "Around the house?"

"Someone was at the window."

On my palm the pills were white, blue, beige, pink: Lasix, Diabinese, Slow-K, Lopressor. "What do you mean?"

She rolled her pills onto the tablecloth and fidgeted with them, made them into a line, then into a circle, then into a line again. I don't know her medicine so well. She's healthy, except for little things. "I mean," she said, "there was someone in the yard last night."

"How do you know?"

"Frank, will you really, please?"

"I'm asking how you know."

"I heard him," she said. She looked down. "I was sitting in the front room and I heard him outside the window."

"You heard him?"

"Yes."

"The front window?"

She got up and went to the sink. This is a trick of hers. At that distance I can't see her face.

"The front window is ten feet off the ground," I said.

"What I know is that there was a man out there last night, right outside the glass." She walked out of the kitchen.

"Let's check," I called after her. I walked into the living room, and when I got there she was looking out the window.

"What is it?"

She was peering out at an angle. All I could see was snow, blue-white.

"Footprints," she said.

I built the house we live in with my two hands. That was forty-nine years ago, when, in my foolishness and crude want of learning, everything I didn't know seemed like a promise. I learned to build a house and then I built one. There are copper fixtures on the pipes, sanded edges on the struts and queen posts. Now, a half-century later, the floors are flat as a billiard table but the man who laid them needs two hands to pick up a woodscrew. This is the diabetes. My feet are gone also. I look down at them and see two black shapes when I walk, things I can't feel. Black clubs. No connection with the ground. If I didn't look, I could go to sleep with my shoes on.

Life takes its toll, and soon the body gives up completely. But it gives up the parts first. This sugar in the blood: God says to me: "Frank Manlius— codger, man of prevarication and half-truth—I shall take your life from you, as from all men. But first—" But first! Clouds in the eyeball, a heart that makes noise, feet cold as uncooked roast. And Francine, beauty that she was—now I see not much more than the dark line of her brow and the intersections of her body: mouth and nose, neck and shoulders. Her smells have changed over the years so that I don't know what's her own anymore and what's powder.

We have two children, but they're gone now too, with children of their own. We have a house, some furniture, small savings to speak of. How Francine spends her day I don't know. This is the sad truth, my confession. I am gone past nightfall. She wakes early with me and is awake when I return, but beyond this I know almost nothing of her life.

I myself spend my days at the aquarium. I've told Francine something else, of course, that I'm part of a volunteer service of retired men, that we spend our days setting young businesses afoot: "Immigrants," I told her early on, "newcomers to the land." I said it was difficult work. In the evenings I could invent stories, but I don't, and Francine doesn't ask.

I am home by nine or ten. Ticket stubs from the aquarium fill my coat pocket. Most of the day I watch the big sea animals—porpoises, sharks, a manatee—turn their saltwater loops. I come late morning and move a chair up close. They are waiting to eat then. Their bodies skim the cool glass, full of strange magnifications. I think, if it is possible, that they are beginning to know me: this man—hunched at the shoulder, cataractic of eye, breathing through water himself—this man who sits and watches. I do not pity them. At lunchtime I buy coffee and sit in one of the hotel lobbies or in the cafeteria next door, and I read poems. Browning, Whitman, Eliot. This is my secret. It is night when I return home. Francine is at the table, four feet across from my seat, the width of two dropleaves. Our medicine is in cups. There have been three Presidents since I held her in my arms.

The cafeteria moves the men along, old or young, who come to get away from the cold. A half-hour for a cup, they let me sit. Then the manager is at my table. He is nothing but polite. I buy a pastry then, something small. He knows me—I have seen him nearly every day for months now—and by his slight limp I know he is a man of mercy. But business is business.

"What are you reading?" he asks me as he wipes the table with a wet cloth. He touches the saltshaker, nudges the napkins in their holder. I know what this means.

"I'll take a cranberry roll," I say. He flicks the cloth and turns back to the counter.

This is what:

> Shall I say, I have gone at dusk through narrow streets
> And watched the smoke that rises from the pipes
> Of lonely men in shirt-sleeves, leaning out of windows?

Through the magnifier glass the words come forward, huge, two by two. With spectacles, everything is twice enlarged. Still, though, I am slow to read it. In a half-hour I am finished, could not read more, even if I bought another roll. The boy at the register greets me, smiles when I reach him. "What are you reading today?" he asks, counting the change.

The books themselves are small and fit in the inside pockets of my coat. I put one in front of each breast, then walk back to see the fish some more. These are the fish I know: the gafftopsail pompano, sixgill shark, the starry flounder with its upturned eyes, queerly migrated. He rests half-submerged in sand. His scales are platey and flat-hued. Of everything upward he is wary, of the silvery seabass and the bluefin tuna that pass above him in the region of light and open water. For a life he lies on the bottom of the tank. I look at him. His eyes are dull. They are ugly and an aberration. Above us the bony fishes wheel at the tank's corners. I lean forward to the glass. "*Platichthys stellatus*," I say to him. The caudal fin stirs. Sand moves and re-settles, and I see the black and yellow stripes. "Flatfish," I whisper, "we are, you and I, observers of this life."

"A man on our lawn," I say a few nights later in bed.
"Not just that."
I breathe in, breathe out, look up at the ceiling. "What else?"
"When you were out last night he came back."
"He came back."
"Yes."
"What did he do?"

"Looked in at me."

Later, in the early night, when the lights of cars are still passing and the walked dogs still jingle their collar chains out front, I get up quickly from bed and step into the hall. I move fast because this is still possible in short bursts and with concentration. The bed sinks once, then rises. I am on the landing and then downstairs without Francine waking. I stay close to the staircase joists.

In the kitchen I take out my almost blank sheets and set them on the counter. I write standing up because I want to take more than an animal's pose. For me this is futile, but I stand anyway. The page will be blank when I finish. This I know. The dreams I compose are the dreams of others, remembered bits of verse. Songs of greater men than I. In months I have written few more than a hundred words. The pages are stacked, sheets of different sizes.

If I could

one says.

It has never seemed

says another. I stand and shift them in and out. They are mostly blank, sheets from months of nights. But this doesn't bother me. What I have is patience.

Francine knows nothing of the poetry. She's a simple girl, toast and butter. I myself am hardly the man for it: forty years selling (anything—steel piping, heater elements, dried bananas). Didn't read a book except one on sales. Think victory, the book said. Think sale. It's a young man's bag of apples, though; young men in pants that nip at the waist. Ten years ago I left the Buick in the company lot and walked home, dye in my hair, cotton rectangles in the shoulders of my coat. Francine was in the house that afternoon also, the way she is now. When I retired we bought a camper and went on a trip. A traveling salesman retires, so he goes on a trip. Forty miles out of town the folly appeared to me, big as a balloon. To Francine, too. "Frank," she said in the middle of a bend, a prophet turning to me, the camper pushing sixty and rocking in the wind, trucks to our left and right big as trains—"Frank," she said, "these roads must be familiar to you."

So we sold the camper at a loss and a man who'd spent forty years at highway speed looked around for something to do before he died. The first poem I read was in a book on a table in a waiting room. My eyeglasses made half-sense of things.

THESE
are the desolate, dark weeks

I read

when nature in its barrenness
equals the stupidity of man.

Gloom, I thought, and nothing more, but then I reread the words, and suddenly there I was, hunched and wheezing, bald as a trout, and tears were in my eye. I don't know where they came from.

In the morning an officer visits. He has muscles, mustache, skin red from the cold. He leans against the door frame.

"Can you describe him?" he says.

"It's always dark," says Francine.

"Anything about him?"

"I'm an old woman. I can see that he wears glasses."

"What kind of glasses?"

"Black."

"Dark glasses?"

"Black glasses."

"At a particular time?"

"Always when Frank is away."

"Your husband has never been here when he's come?"

"Never."

"I see." He looks at me. This look can mean several things, perhaps that he thinks Francine is imagining. "But never at a particular time?"

"No."

"Well," he says. Outside on the porch his partner is stamping his feet. "Well," he says again. "We'll have a look." He turns, replaces his cap, heads out to the snowy steps. The door closes. I hear him say something outside.

"Last night—" Francine says. She speaks in the dark. "Last night I heard him on the side of the house."

We are in bed. Outside, on the sill, snow has been building since morning.

"You heard the wind."

"Frank." She sits up, switches on the lamp, tilts her head toward the window. Through a ceiling and two walls I can hear the ticking of our kitchen clock.

"I heard him climbing," she says. She has wrapped her arms about her own waist. "He was on the house. I heard him. He went up the drainpipe." She shivers as she says this. "There was no wind. He went up the drainpipe and then I heard him on the porch roof."

"Houses make noise."

"I heard him. There's gravel there."

I imagine the sounds, amplified by hollow walls, rubber heels on timber. I don't say anything. There is an arm's length between us, cold sheet, a space uncrossed since I can remember.

"I have made the mistake in my life of not being interested in enough people," she says then. "If I'd been interested in more people, I wouldn't be alone now."

"Nobody's alone," I say.

"I mean that if I'd made more of an effort with people I would have friends now. I would know the postman and the Giffords and the Kohlers, and we'd be together in this, all of us. We'd sit in each other's living rooms on rainy days and talk about the children. Instead we've kept to ourselves. I'm alone."

"You're not alone," I say.

"Yes, I am." She turns the light off and we are in the dark again. "You're alone, too."

My health has gotten worse. It's slow to set in at this age not the violent shaking grip of death; instead—a slow leak nothing more. A bicycle tire: rimless, thready, worn treadless already and now losing its fatness. A war of attrition. The tall camels of the spirit steering for the desert. One morning I realized I hadn't been warm in a year.

And there are other things that go, too. For instance, I recall with certainty that it was on the 23rd of April, 1945, that, despite German counteroffensives in the Ardennes, Eisenhower's men reached the Elbe; but I cannot remember whether I have visited the savings and loan this week. Also I am unable to produce the name of my neighbor, though I greeted him yesterday in the street. And take, for example, this: I am at a loss to explain whole decades of my life. We have children and photographs, and there is an understanding between Francine and me that bears the weight of nothing less than half a century, but when I gather my memories they seem to fill no more than an hour. Where has my life gone?

It has gone partway to shoddy accumulations. In my wallet are credit cards, a license ten years expired, twenty-three dollars in cash. There is a photograph but it depresses me to look at it, and a poem, half-copied and folded into the billfold. The leather is pocked and has taken on the curve of my thigh. The poem is from Walt Whitman. I copy only what I need.

But of all things to do last, poetry is a barren choice. Deciphering other men's riddles while the world is full of procreation and war. A man should go out swinging an axe. Instead, I shall go out in a coffee shop.

But how can any man leave this world with honor? Despite anything he does, it grows corrupt around him. It fills with locks and sirens. A man walks into a store now and the microwaves announce his entry; when he leaves, they make electronic peeks into his coat pockets, his trousers. Who doesn't feel like a thief? I see a policeman now, any policeman, and I feel a fright. And the things I've done wrong in my life haven't been crimes. Crimes of the heart perhaps, but nothing against the state. My soul may turn black but I can wear white trousers at any meeting of men. Have I loved my wife? At one time, yes—in rages and torrents. I've been covered by the pimples of ecstasy and have rooted in the mud of despair; and I've lived for months, for whole years now, as mindless of Francine as a tree of its mosses.

And this is what kills us, this mindlessness. We sit across the tablecloth now with our medicines between us, little balls and oblongs. We sit, sit. This has become our view of each other, a tableboard apart. We sit.

❧

"Again?" I say.

"Last night."

We are at the table. Francine is making a twisting motion with her fingers. She coughs, brushes her cheek with her forearm, stands suddenly so that the table bumps and my medicines move in the cup.

"Francine," I say.

The half-light of dawn is showing me things outside the window: silhouettes, our maple, the eaves of our neighbor's garage. Francine moves and stands against the glass, hugging her shoulders.

"You're not telling me something," I say.

She sits and makes her pills into a circle again, then into a line. Then she is crying.

I come around the table, but she gets up before I reach her and leaves the kitchen. I stand there. In a moment I hear a drawer open in the living room. She moves things around, then shuts it again. When she returns she sits at the other side of the table. "Sit down," she says. She puts two folded sheets of paper onto the table. "I wasn't hiding them," she says.

"What weren't you hiding?"

"These," she says. "He leaves them."

"He leaves them?"

"They say he loves me."

"Francine."

"They're inside the windows in the morning." She picks one up, unfolds it. Then she reads:

Ah, I remember well (and how can I
But evermore remember well) when first

She pauses, squint-eyed, working her lips. It is a pause of only faint understanding. Then she continues:

Our flame began, when scarce we knew what was
The flame we felt.

When she finishes she refolds the paper precisely. "That's it," she says. "That's one of them."

At the aquarium I sit, circled by glass and, behind it, the senseless eyes of fish. I have never written a word of my own poetry but can recite the verse of others. This is the culmination of a life. *Coryphaena hippurus*, says the plaque on the dolphin's tank, words more beautiful than any of my own. The dolphin circles, circles, approaches with alarming speed, but takes no notice of, if he even sees, my hands. I wave them in front of his tank. What must he think has become of the sea? He turns and his slippery proboscis nudges the glass. I am every part sore from life.

Ah, silver shrine, here will I take my rest
After so many hours of toil and quest,
A famished pilgrim—saved by miracle.

There is nothing noble for either of us here, nothing between us, and no miracles. I am better off drinking coffee. Any fluid refills the blood. The counter boy knows me and later at the café he pours the cup, most of a dollar's worth. Refills are free but my heart hurts if I drink more than one. It hurts no different from a bone, bruised or cracked. This amazes me.

Francine is amazed by other things. She is mystified, thrown beam ends by the romance. She reads me the poems now at breakfast, one by one. I sit. I roll my pills. "Another came last night," she says, and I see her eyebrows rise. "Another this morning." She reads them as if every word is a surprise. Her tongue touches teeth, shows between lips. These lips are dry. She reads:

Kiss me as if you made believe
You were not sure, this eve,
How my face, your flower, had pursed
Its petals up

That night she shows me the windowsill, second story, rimmed with snow, where she finds the poems. We open the glass. We lean into the air. There is ice below us, sheets of it on the trellis, needles hanging from the drainwork.

"Where do you find them?"

"Outside," she says. "Folded, on the lip."

"In the morning?"

"Always in the morning."

"The police should know about this."

"What will they be able to do?"

I step away from the sill. She leans out again, surveying her lands, which are the yard's-width spit of crusted ice along our neighbor's chain link and the three maples out front, now lost their leaves. She peers as if she expects this man to appear. An icy wind comes inside. "Think," she says. "Think. He could come from anywhere."

☙

One night in February, a month after this began, she asks me to stay awake and stand guard until the morning. It is almost spring. The earth has reappeared in patches. During the day, at the borders of yards and driveways, I see glimpses of brown—though I know I could be mistaken. I come home early that night, before dusk, and when darkness falls I move a chair by the window downstairs. I draw apart the outer curtain and raise the shade. Francine brings me a pot of tea. She turns out the light and pauses next to me, and as she does, her hand on the chair's backbrace, I am so struck by the proximity of elements—of the night, of the teapot's heat, of the sounds of water outside—that I consider speaking. I want to ask her what has become of us, what has made our breathed air so sorry now, and loveless. But the timing is wrong and in a moment she turns and climbs the stairs. I look out into the night. Later, I hear the closet shut, then our bed creak.

There is nothing to see outside, nothing to hear. This I know. I let hours pass. Behind the window I imagine fish moving down to greet me: broomtail grouper, surfperch, sturgeon with their prehistoric rows of scutes. It is almost possible to see them. The night is full of shapes and bits of light. In it the moon rises, losing the colors of the horizon, so that by early morning it is high and pale. Frost has made a ring around it.

A ringed moon above, and I am thinking back on things. What have I regretted in my life? Plenty of things, mistakes enough to fill the car show-room, then a good deal of the back lot. I've been a man of gains and losses. What gains? My marriage, certainly, though it has been no knee-buckling windfall but more like a split decision in the end, a stock risen a few points since bought. I've certainly enjoyed certain things about the world, too. These are things gone over and over again by the writers and probably enjoyed by everybody who ever lived. Most of them involve air. Early morning air, air after a rainstorm, air through a car window. Sometimes I think the cerebrum is wasted and all we really need is the lower brain, which I've been told is what makes the lungs breathe and the heart beat and what lets us smell pleasant things. What about the poetry? That's another split decision, maybe going the other way if I really made a tally. It's made me melancholy in old age, sad when if I'd stuck with motor homes and the national league standings I don't think I would have been rooting around in regret and doubt at this point. Nothing wrong with sadness, but this is not the real thing—not the death of a child but the feelings of a college student reading Don Quixote on a warm afternoon before going out to the lake.

Now, with Francine upstairs, I wait for a night prowler. He will not appear. This I know, but the window glass is illblown and makes moving shadows anyway, shapes that change in the wind's rattle. I look out and despite myself am afraid.

Before me, the night unrolls. Now the tree leaves turn yellow in moonshine. By two or three, Francine sleeps, but I get up anyway and change into my coat and hat. The books weigh against my chest. I don gloves, scarf, galoshes. Then I climb the stairs and go into our bedroom, where she is sleeping. On the far side of the bed I see her white hair and beneath the blankets the uneven heave of her chest. I watch the bedcovers rise. She is probably dreaming at this moment. Though we have shared this bed for most of a lifetime I cannot guess what her dreams are about. I step next to her and touch the sheets where they lie across her neck.

"Wake up," I whisper. I touch her cheek, and her eyes open. I know this though I cannot really see them, just the darkness of their sockets.

"Is he there?"

"No."

"Then what's the matter?"

"Nothing's the matter," I say. "But I'd like to go for a walk."

"You've been outside," she says. "You saw him, didn't you?"

"I've been at the window."

"Did you see him?"

"No. There's no one there."

"Then why do you want to walk?" In a moment she is sitting aside the bed, her feet in slippers. "We don't ever walk," she says.

I am warm in all my clothing. "I know we don't," I answer. I turn my arms out, open my hands toward her. "But I would like to. I would like to walk in air that is so new and cold."

She peers up at me. "I haven't been drinking," I say. I bend at the waist, and though my head spins, I lean forward enough so that the effect is of a bow. "Will you come with me?" I whisper. "Will you be queen of this crystal night?" I recover from my bow, and when I look up again she has risen from the bed, and in another moment she has dressed herself in her wool robe and is walking ahead of me to the stairs.

Outside, the ice is treacherous. Snow has begun to fall and our galoshes squeak and slide, but we stay on the plowed walkway long enough to leave our block and enter a part of the neighborhood where I have never been. Ice hangs from the lamps. We pass unfamiliar houses and unfamiliar trees, street signs I have never seen, and as we walk the night begins to change. It is becoming liquor. The snow is banked on either side of the walk, plowed into hillocks at the corners. My hands are warming from the exertion. They are the hands of a younger man now, someone else's fingers in my gloves. They tingle. We take ten minutes to cover a block but as we move through this neighborhood my ardor mounts. A car approaches and I wave, a boatman's salute, because here we are together on these rare and empty seas. We are nighttime travelers. He flashes his headlamps as he passes, and this fills me to the gullet with celebration and bravery. The night sings to us. I am Bluebeard now, Lindbergh, Genghis Khan.

No, I am not.

I am an old man. My blood is dark from hypoxia, my breaths singsong from disease. It is only the frozen night that is splendid. In it we walk, stepping slowly, bent forward. We take steps the length of table forks. Francine holds my elbow.

I have mean secrets and small dreams, no plans greater than where to buy groceries and what rhymes to read next, and by the time we reach our porch again my foolishness has subsided. My knees and elbows ache. They ache with a mortal ache, tired flesh, the cartilage gone sandy with time. I don't have the heart for dreams. We undress in the hallway, ice in the ends of our hair, our coats stiff from cold. Francine turns down the thermostat. Then we go upstairs and she gets into her side of the bed and I get into mine.

It is dark. We lie there for some time, and then, before dawn, I know she is asleep. It is cold in our bedroom. As I listen to her breathing I know my life is coming to an end. I cannot warm myself. What I would like to tell my wife is this:

What the
imagination
seizes
as beauty must be truth. What holds you
to what you see of me is
that grasp alone.

But I do not say anything. Instead I roll in the bed, reach across, and touch her, and because she is surprised she turns to me.

When I kiss her the lips are dry, cracking against mine, unfamiliar as the ocean floor. But then the lips give. They part. I am inside her mouth, and there, still, hidden from the world, as if ruin had forgotten a part, it is wet—Lord! I have the feeling of a miracle. Her tongue comes forward. I do not know myself then, what man I am, who I lie with in embrace. I can barely remember her beauty. She touches my chest and I bite lightly on her lip, spread moisture to her cheek and then kiss there. She makes something like a sigh. "Frank," she says. "Frank." We are lost now in seas and deserts. My hand finds her fingers and grips them, bone and tendon, fragile things.

13

The Ship Pounding

& *Donald Hall*

Each morning I made my way
among gangways, elevators,
and nurses' pods to Jane's room
to interrogate grave helpers
who had tended her all night
like the ship's massive engines
kept its propellers turning.
Week after week, I sat by her bed
with black coffee and the *Globe*.
The passengers on this voyage
wore masks or cannulae
or dangled devices that dripped
chemicals into their wrists,
but I believed that the ship
travelled to a harbor
of breakfast, work, and love.
I wrote: "When the infusions
are infused entirely, bone
marrow restored and lymphoblasts
remitted, I will take my wife,
as bald as Michael Jordan,
home to our dog and day."
Months later these words turn up
among papers on my desk at home,
as I listen to hear Jane call
for help, or speak in delirium,

waiting to make the agitated
drive to Emergency again,
for re-admission to the huge
vessel that heaves water month
after month, without leaving
port, without moving a knot,
without arrival or destination,
its great engines pounding.

14

The Sick Wife

❦ Jane Kenyon

The sick wife stayed in the car
while he bought a few groceries.
Not yet fifty,
she had learned what it's like
not to be able to button a button.

It was the middle of the day—
and so only mothers with small children
or retired couples
stepped through the muddy parking lot.

Dry cleaning swung and gleamed on hangers
in the cars of the prosperous.
How easily they moved—
with such freedom,
even the old and relatively infirm.

The windows began to steam up.
The cars on either side of her
pulled away so briskly
that it made her sick at heart.

15

Alzheimer's: The Wife

FOR RENÉE MAUGER

✿ *C. K. Williams*

She answers the bothersome telephone, takes the
    message, forgets the message, forgets who called.
One of their daughters, her husband guesses: the
    one with the dogs, the babies, the boy Jed?
Yes, perhaps, but how tell which, how tell anything
    when all the name tags have been lost or switched,
when all the lonely flowers of sense and memory
    bloom and die now in adjacent bites of time?
Sometimes her own face will suddenly appear with
    terrifying inappropriateness before her in a mirror.
She knows that if she's patient, its gaze will break,
    demurely, decorously, like a well-taught child's,
it will turn from her as though it were embarrassed
    by the secrets of this awful hide-and-seek.
If she forgets, though, and glances back again, it
    will still be in there, furtively watching, crying.

16

Alzheimer's: The Husband

FOR JEAN MAUGER

& C. K. Williams

He'd been a clod, he knew, yes, always aiming toward
    his vision of the good life, always acting on it.
He knew he'd been unconscionably self-centered, had
    indulged himself with his undreamed-of good fortune,
but he also knew that the single-mindedness with which
    he'd attended to his passions, needs and whims,
and which must have seemed to others the grossest sort
    of egotism, was also what was really at the base
of how he'd almost offhandedly worked out the
    intuitions and moves which had brought him here,
and this wasn't all that different: to spend his long-
    anticipated retirement learning to cook
clean house, dress her, even to apply her makeup,
    wasn't any sort of secular saintliness—
that would be belittling—it was just the next
    necessity he saw himself as being called to.

17

The Bear Came Over
the Mountain

 Alice Munro

Fiona lived in her parents' house, in the town where she and Grant went to university. It was a big, bay-windowed house that seemed to Grant both luxurious and disorderly, with rugs crooked on the floors and cup rings bitten into the table varnish. Her mother was Icelandic—a powerful woman with a froth of white hair and indignant far-left politics. The father was an important cardiologist, revered around the hospital but happily subservient at home, where he would listen to his wife's strange tirades with an absent-minded smile. Fiona had her own little car and a pile of cashmere sweaters, but she wasn't in a sorority, and her mother's political activity was probably the reason. Not that she cared. Sororities were a joke to her, and so was politics—though she liked to play "The Four Insurgent Generals" on the phonograph, and sometimes also the "Internationale," very loud, if there was a guest she thought she could make nervous. A curly-haired gloomy-looking foreigner was courting her—she said he was a Visigoth—and so were two or three quite respectable and uneasy young interns. She made fun of them all and of Grant as well. She would drolly repeat some of his small-town phrases. He thought maybe she was joking when she proposed to him, on a cold bright day on the beach at Port Stanley. Sand was stinging their faces and the waves delivered crashing loads of gravel at their feet.

"Do you think it would be fun—" Fiona shouted. "Do you think it would be fun if we got married?"

He took her up on it, he shouted yes. He wanted never to be away from her. She had the spark of life.

Just before they left their house Fiona noticed a mark on the kitchen floor. It came from the cheap black house shoes she had been wearing earlier in the day.

"I thought they'd quit doing that," she said in a tone of ordinary annoyance and perplexity, rubbing at the gray smear that looked as if it had been made by a greasy crayon.

She remarked that she'd never have to do this again, since she wasn't taking those shoes with her.

"I guess I'll be dressed up all the time," she said. "Or semi-dressed up. It'll be sort of like in a hotel."

She rinsed out the rag she'd been using and hung it on the rack inside the door under the sink. Then she put on her golden-brown, fur-collared ski jacket, over a white turtleneck sweater and tailored fawn slacks. She was a tall, narrow-shouldered woman, seventy years old but still upright and trim, with long legs and long feet, delicate wrists and ankles, and tiny, almost comical-looking ears. Her hair that was as light as milkweed fluff had gone from pale blond to white somehow without Grant's noticing exactly when, and she still wore it down to her shoulders, as her mother had done. (That was the thing that had alarmed Grant's own mother, a small-town widow who worked as a doctor's receptionist. The long white hair on Fiona's mother, even more than the state of the house, had told her all she needed to know about attitudes and politics.) But otherwise Fiona, with her fine bones and small sapphire eyes, was nothing like her mother. She had a slightly crooked mouth, which she emphasized now with red lipstick—usually the last thing she did before she left the house.

She looked just like herself on this day—direct and vague as in fact she was, sweet and ironic.

Over a year ago, Grant had started noticing so many little yellow notes stuck up all over the house. That was not entirely new. Fiona had always written things down—the title of a book she'd heard mentioned on the radio or the jobs she wanted to make sure she got done that day. Even her morning schedule was written down. He found it mystifying and touching in its precision: "7 a.m. yoga. 7:30–7:45 teeth face hair. 7:45–8:15 walk. 8:15 Grant and breakfast."

The new notes were different. Stuck onto the kitchen drawers—Cutlery, Dishtowels, Knives. Couldn't she just open the drawers and see what was inside?

Worse things were coming. She went to town and phoned Grant from a booth to ask him how to drive home. She went for her usual walk across the field into the woods and came home by the fence line—a very long way round. She said that she'd counted on fences always taking you somewhere.

It was hard to figure out. She'd said that about fences as if it were a joke, and she had remembered the phone number without any trouble.

"I don't think it's anything to worry about," she said. "I expect I'm just losing my mind."

He asked if she had been taking sleeping pills.

"If I am I don't remember," she said. Then she said she was sorry to sound so flippant. "I'm sure I haven't been taking anything. Maybe I should be. Maybe vitamins."

Vitamins didn't help. She would stand in doorways trying to figure out where she was going. She forgot to turn on the burner under the vegetables or put water in the coffeemaker. She asked Grant when they'd moved to this house.

"Was it last year or the year before?"

"It was twelve years ago," he said.

"That's shocking."

"She's always been a bit like this," Grant said to the doctor. He tried without success to explain how Fiona's surprise and apologies now seemed somehow like routine courtesy, not quite concealing a private amusement. As if she'd stumbled on some unexpected adventure. Or begun playing a game that she hoped he would catch on to.

"Yes, well," the doctor said. "It might be selective at first. We don't know, do we? Till we see the pattern of the deterioration, we really can't say."

In a while it hardly mattered what label was put on it. Fiona, who no longer went shopping alone, disappeared from the supermarket while Grant had his back turned. A policeman picked her up as she was walking down the middle of the road, blocks away. He asked her name and she answered readily. Then he asked her the name of the Prime Minister.

"If you don't know that, young man, you really shouldn't be in such a re-sponsible job."

He laughed. But then she made the mistake of asking if he'd seen Boris and Natasha. These were the now dead Russian wolfhounds she had adopted many years ago, as a favor to a friend, then devoted herself to for the rest of their lives. Her taking them over might have coincided with the discovery that she was not likely to have children. Something about her tubes being blocked, or twisted—Grant could not remember now. He had always avoided thinking about all that female apparatus. Or it might have been after her mother died. The dogs' long legs and silky hair, their narrow, gentle, intransigent faces made a fine match for her when she took them out for walks. And Grant himself, in those days, landing his first job at the university (his father-in-law's money welcome there in spite of the political taint), might have seemed to some people to have been picked up on another of Fiona's eccentric whims, and groomed and tended and favored—though, fortunately, he didn't understand this until much later.

There was a rule that nobody could be admitted to Meadowlake during the month of December. The holiday season had so many emotional pitfalls. So they made the twenty-minute drive in January. Before they reached the highway the country road dipped through a swampy hollow now completely frozen over.

Fiona said, "Oh, remember."

Grant said, "I was thinking about that, too."

"Only it was in the moonlight," she said.

She was talking about the time that they had gone out skiing at night under the full moon and over the black-striped snow, in this place that you could get into only in the depths of winter. They had heard the branches cracking in the cold.

If she could remember that, so vividly and correctly, could there really be so much the matter with her? It was all he could do not to turn around and drive home.

There was another rule that the supervisor explained to him. New residents were not to be visited during the first thirty days. Most people needed that time to get settled in. Before the rule had been put in place, there had been pleas and tears and tantrums, even from those who had come in willingly. Around the third or fourth day they would start lamenting and begging to be taken home. And some relatives could be susceptible to that, so you would have people being carted home who would not get on there any better than they had before. Six months or sometimes only a few weeks later, the whole upsetting hassle would have to be gone through again.

"Whereas we find," the supervisor said, "we find that if they're left on their own the first month they usually end up happy as clams."

They had in fact gone over to Meadowlake a few times several years ago to visit Mr. Farquhar, the old bachelor farmer who had been their neighbor. He had lived by himself in a drafty brick house unaltered since the early years of the century, except for the addition of a refrigerator and a television set. Now, just as Mr. Farquhar's house was gone, replaced by a gimcrack sort of castle that was the weekend home of some people from Toronto, the old Meadowlake was gone, though it had dated only from the fifties. The new building was a spacious, vaulted place, whose air was faintly, pleasantly pine-scented. Profuse and genuine greenery sprouted out of giant crocks in the hallways.

Nevertheless, it was the old Meadowlake that Grant found himself picturing Fiona in, during the long month he had to get through without seeing her. He phoned every day and hoped to get the nurse whose name was Kristy. She seemed a little amused at his constancy, but she would give him a fuller report than any other nurse he got stuck with.

Fiona had caught a cold the first week, she said, but that was not unusual for newcomers. "Like when your kids start school," Kristy said. "There's a whole bunch of new germs they're exposed to and for a while they just catch everything."

Then the cold got better. She was off the antibiotics and she didn't seem as confused as she had been when she came in. (This was the first Grant had heard about either the antibiotics or the confusion.) Her appetite was pretty good and she seemed to enjoy sitting in the sunroom. And she was making some friends, Kristy said.

If anybody phoned, he let the machine pick up. The people they saw socially, occasionally, were not close neighbors but people who lived around the country, who were retired, as they were, and who often went away without notice. They would imagine that he and Fiona were away on some such trip at present.

Grant skied for exercise. He skied around and around in the field behind the house as the sun went down and left the sky pink over a countryside that seemed to be bound by waves of blue-edged ice. Then he came back to the darkening house, turning the television news on while he made his supper. They had usually prepared supper together. One of them made the drinks and the other the fire, and they talked about his work (he was writing a study of legendary Norse wolves and particularly of the great wolf Fenrir, which swallows up Odin at the end of the world) and about whatever Fiona was reading and what they had been thinking during their close but separate day. This was their time of liveliest intimacy, though there was also, of course, the five or ten minutes of physical sweetness just after they got into bed—something that did not often end in sex but reassured them that sex was not over yet.

In a dream he showed a letter to one of his colleagues. The letter was from the roommate of a girl he had not thought of for a while and was sanctimonious and hostile, threatening in a whining way. The girl herself was someone he had parted from decently and it seemed unlikely that she would want to make a fuss, let alone try to kill herself, which was what the letter was elaborately trying to tell him she had done.

He had thought of the colleague as a friend. He was one of those husbands who had been among the first to throw away their neckties and leave home to spend every night on a floor mattress with a bewitching young mistress—coming to their offices, their classes, bedraggled and smelling of dope and incense. But now he took a dim view. "I wouldn't laugh," he said to Grant—who did not think he had been laughing. "And if I were you I'd try to prepare Fiona."

So Grant went off to find Fiona in Meadowlake—the old Meadowlake—and got into a lecture hall instead. Everybody was waiting there for him to teach his class. And sitting in the last, highest row was a flock of cold-eyed young women all in black robes, all in mourning, who never took their bitter stares off him, and pointedly did not write down, or care about, anything he was saying.

Fiona was in the first row, untroubled. "Oh phooey," she said. "Girls that age are always going around talking about how they'll kill themselves."

He hauled himself out of the dream, took pills, and set about separating what was real from what was not.

There *had* been a letter, and the word "rat" had appeared in black paint on his office door, and Fiona, on being told that a girl had suffered from a bad crush on him, had said pretty much what she said in the dream. The colleague hadn't come into it, and nobody had committed suicide. Grant hadn't been disgraced. In fact, he had got off easy when you thought of what might have happened just a couple of years later. But word got around. Cold shoulders became conspicuous. They had few Christmas invitations and spent New Year's Eve alone. Grant got drunk, and without its being required of him—also, thank God, without making the error of a confession—he promised Fiona a new life.

Nowhere had there been any acknowledgment that the life of a philanderer (if that was what Grant had to call himself—he who had not had half as many conquests as the man who had reproached him in his dream) involved acts of generosity, and even sacrifice. Many times he had catered to a woman's pride, to her fragility, by offering more affection—or a rougher passion—than anything he really felt. All so that he could now find himself accused of wounding and exploiting and destroying self-esteem. And of deceiving Fiona—as, of course, he had. But would it have been better if he had done as others had done with their wives, and left her? He had never thought of such a thing. He had never stopped making love to Fiona. He had not stayed away from her for a single night. No making up elaborate stories in order to spend a weekend in San Francisco or in a tent on Manitoulin Island. He had gone easy on the dope and the drink, and he had continued to publish papers, serve on committees, make progress in his career. He had never had any intention of throwing over work and marriage and taking to the country to practice carpentry or keep bees.

But something like that had happened, after all. He had taken early retirement with a reduced pension. Fiona's father had died, after some bewildered and stoical time alone in the big house, and Fiona had inherited both that property and the farmhouse where her father had grown up, in the country near Georgian Bay.

It was a new life. He and Fiona worked on the house. They got cross-country skis. They were not very sociable but they gradually made some friends. There were no more hectic flirtations. No bare female toes creeping up under a man's pants leg at a dinner party. No more loose wives.

Just in time, Grant was able to think, when the sense of injustice had worn down. The feminists and perhaps the sad silly girl herself and his cowardly so-called friends had pushed him out just in time. Out of a life that was in fact getting to be more trouble than it was worth. And that might eventually have cost him Fiona.

On the morning of the day when he was to go back to Meadowlake, for the first visit, Grant woke early. He was full of a solemn tingling, as in the old days on the morning of his first planned meeting with a new woman. The feeling was not precisely sexual. (Later, when the meetings had become routine, that was all it was.) There was an expectation of discovery, almost a spiritual expansion. Also timidity, humility, alarm.

There had been a thaw. Plenty of snow was left, but the dazzling hard landscape of earlier winter had crumbled. These pocked heaps under a gray sky looked like refuse in the fields. In the town near Meadowlake he found a florist's shop and bought a large bouquet. He had never presented flowers to Fiona before. Or to anyone else. He entered the building feeling like a hopeless lover or a guilty husband in a cartoon.

"Wow. Narcissus this early," Kristy said. "You must've spent a fortune." She went along the hall ahead of him and snapped on the light in a sort of pantry, where she searched for a vase. She was a heavy young woman who looked as if she had given up on her looks in every department except her hair. That was blond and voluminous. All the puffed-up luxury of a cocktail waitress's style, or a stripper's, on top of such a workaday face and body.

"There now," she said, and nodded him down the hall. "Name's right on the door."

So it was, on a nameplate decorated with bluebirds. He wondered whether to knock, and did, then opened the door and called her name.

She wasn't there. The closet door was closed, the bed smoothed.

Nothing on the bedside table, except a box of Kleenex and a glass of water. Not a single photograph or picture of any kind, not a book or a magazine. Perhaps you had to keep those in a cupboard.

He went back to the nurses' station. Kristy said, "No?" with a surprise that he thought perfunctory. He hesitated, holding the flowers. She said, "O.K., O.K.—let's set the bouquet down here." Sighing, as if he were a backward child on his first day at school, she led him down the hall toward a large central space with skylights which seemed to be a general meeting area. Some people were sitting along the walls, in easy chairs, others at tables in the middle of the carpeted floor. None of them looked too bad. Old—some of them incapacitated enough to need wheelchairs—but decent. There had been some unnerving sights when he and Fiona visited Mr. Farquhar. Whiskers on old women's chins, somebody with a bulged-out eye like a rotted plum. Dribblers, head wagglers, mad chatterers. Now it looked as if there'd been some weeding out of the worst cases.

"See?" said Kristy in a softer voice. "You just go up and say hello and try not to startle her. Just go ahead."

He saw Fiona in profile, sitting close up to one of the card tables, but not playing. She looked a little puffy in the face, the flab on one cheek hiding the corner of her mouth, in a way it hadn't done before. She was watching the play of the man she sat closest to. He held his cards tilted so that she could see them. When Grant got near the table she looked up. They all looked up—all the players at the table looked up, with displeasure. Then they immediately looked down at their cards, as if to ward off any intrusion.

But Fiona smiled her lopsided, abashed, sly, and charming smile and pushed back her chair and came round to him, putting her fingers to her mouth.

"Bridge," she whispered. "Deadly serious. They're quite rabid about it." She drew him toward the coffee table, chatting. "I can remember being like that for a while at college. My friends and I would cut class and sit in the common room and smoke and play like cutthroats. Can I get you anything? A cup of tea? I'm afraid the coffee isn't up to much here."

Grant never drank tea.

He could not throw his arms around her. Something about her voice and smile, familiar as they were, something about the way she seemed to be guarding the players from him—as well as him from their displeasure—made that impossible.

"I brought you some flowers," he said. "I thought they'd do to brighten up your room. I went to your room but you weren't there."

"Well, no," she said. "I'm here." She glanced back at the table.

Grant said, "You've made a new friend." He nodded toward the man she'd been sitting next to. At this moment that man looked up at Fiona and she turned, either because of what Grant had said or because she felt the look at her back.

"It's just Aubrey," she said. "The funny thing is I knew him years and years ago. He worked in the store. The hardware store where my grandpa used to shop. He and I were always kidding around and he couldn't get up the nerve to ask me out. Till the very last weekend and he took me to a ballgame. But when it was over my grandpa showed up to drive me home. I was up visiting for the summer. Visiting my grandparents—they lived on a farm."

"Fiona. I know where your grandparents lived. It's where we live. Lived."

"Really?" she said, not paying her full attention because the card-player was sending her his look, which was one not of supplication but of command. He was a man of about Grant's age, or a little older. Thick coarse white hair fell over his forehead and his skin was leathery but pale, yellowish-white like an old wrinkled-up kid glove. His long face was dig-nified and melancholy and he had something of the beauty of a power-ful, discouraged, elderly horse. But where Fiona was concerned he was not discouraged.

"I better go back," Fiona said, a blush spotting her newly fattened face. "He thinks he can't play without me sitting there. It's silly, I hardly know the game anymore. If I leave you now, you can entertain yourself? It must all seem strange to you but you'll be surprised how soon you get used to it. You'll get to know who everybody is. Except that some of them are pretty well off in the clouds, you know—you can't expect them all to get to know who you are."

She slipped back into her chair and said something into Aubrey's ear. She tapped her fingers across the back of his hand.

Grant went in search of Kristy and met her in the hall. She was pushing a cart with pitchers of apple juice and grape juice.

"Well?" she said.

Grant said, "Does she even know who I am?" He could not decide. She could have been playing a joke. It would not be unlike her. She had given herself away by that little pretense at the end, talking to him as if she thought perhaps he was a new resident. If it was a pretense.

Kristy said, "You just caught her at sort of a bad moment. Involved in the game."

"She's not even playing," he said.

"Well, but her friend's playing. Aubrey."

"So who is Aubrey?"

"That's who he is. Aubrey. Her friend. Would you like a juice?"

Grant shook his head.

"Oh look," said Kristy. "They get these attachments. That takes over for a while. Best buddy sort of thing. It's kind of a phase."

"You mean she really might not know who I am?"

"She might not. Not today. Then tomorrow—you never know, do you? You'll see the way it is, once you've been coming here for a while. You'll learn not to take it all so serious. Learn to take it day by day."

Day by day. But things really didn't change back and forth and he didn't get used to the way they were. Fiona was the one who seemed to get used to him, but only as some persistent visitor who took a special interest in her. Or perhaps even as a nuisance who must be prevented, according to her old rules of courtesy, from realizing that he was one. She treated him with a distracted, social sort of kindness that was successful in keeping him from asking the most obvious, the most necessary question: did she remember him as her husband of nearly fifty years? He got the impression that she would be embarrassed by such a question—embarrassed not for herself but for him.

Kristy told him that Aubrey had been the local representative of a company that sold weed killer "and all that kind of stuff" to farmers. And then when he was not very old or even retired, she said, he had suffered some unusual kind of damage.

"His wife is the one takes care of him, usually at home. She just put him in here on temporary care so she could get a break. Her sister wanted her to go to Florida. See, she's had a hard time, you wouldn't ever have expected a man like him—they just went on a holiday somewhere and he got something, like some bug that gave him a terrible high fever? And it put him in a coma and left him like he is now."

Most afternoons the pair could be found at the card table. Aubrey had large, thick-fingered hands. It was difficult for him to manage his cards. Fiona shuffled and dealt for him and sometimes moved quickly to straighten a card that seemed to be slipping from his grasp. Grant would watch from across the room her darting move and quick laughing apology. He could see Aubrey's husbandly frown as a wisp of her hair touched his cheek. Aubrey preferred to ignore her, as long as she stayed close.

But let her smile her greeting at Grant, let her push back her chair and get up to offer him tea—showing that she had accepted his right to be there—and Aubrey's face took on its look of sombre consternation. He would let the cards slide from his fingers and fall on the floor to spoil the game. And Fiona then had to get busy and put things right.

If Fiona and Aubrey weren't at the bridge table they might be walking along the halls, Aubrey hanging on to the railing with one hand and clutching Fiona's arm or shoulder with the other. The nurses thought that it was a marvel, the way she had got him out of his wheelchair. Though for longer trips—to the conservatory at one end of the building or the television room at the other—the wheelchair was called for.

In the conservatory, the pair would find themselves a seat among the most lush and thick and tropical-looking plants—a bower, if you liked. Grant stood nearby, on occasion, on the other side of the greenery, listening. Mixed in with the rustle of the leaves and the sound of plashing water was Fiona's soft talk and her laughter. Then some sort of chortle. Aubrey could talk, though his voice probably didn't sound as it used to. He seemed to say something now—a couple of thick syllables.

Take care. He's here. My love.

Grant made an effort, and cut his visits down to Wednesdays and Saturdays. Saturdays had a holiday bustle and tension. Families arrived in clusters. Mothers were usually in charge; they were the ones who kept the conversation afloat. Men seemed cowed, teen-agers affronted. No children or grandchildren appeared to visit Aubrey, and since they could not play cards—the tables being taken over for ice-cream parties—he and Fiona stayed clear of the Saturday parade. The conservatory was far too popular then for any of their intimate conversations. Those might be going on, of course, behind Fiona's closed door. Grant could not manage to knock when he found it closed, though he stood there for some time staring at the Disney-style nameplate with an intense, a truly malignant dislike.

Or they might be in Aubrey's room. But he did not know where that was. The more he explored this place the more corridors and seating spaces and ramps he discovered, and in his wanderings he was still apt to get lost. One Saturday he looked out a window and saw Fiona—it had to be her—wheeling Aubrey along one of the paved paths now cleared of snow and ice. She was wearing a silly wool hat and a jacket with swirls of blue and purple, the sort of thing he had seen on local women at the supermarket. It must be that they didn't bother to sort out the wardrobes of the women who were roughly the same size and counted on the women not to recognize their own clothes anyway. They had cut her hair, too. They had cut away her angelic halo.

On a Wednesday, when everything was more normal and card games were going on again and the women in the Crafts Room were making silk flowers or costumed dolls—and when Aubrey and Fiona were again in evidence, so that it was possible for Grant to have one of his brief and friendly and maddening conversations with his wife—he said to her, "Why did they chop off your hair?"

Fiona put her hands up to her head, to check.

"Why—I never missed it," she said.

When Grant had first started teaching Anglo-Saxon and Nordic literature he got the regular sort of students in his classes. But after a few years he noticed a change. Married women had started going back to school. Not with the idea of qualifying for a better job, or for any job, but simply to give themselves something more interesting to think about than their usual housework and hobbies. To enrich their lives. And perhaps it followed naturally that the men who taught them these things became part of the enrichment, that these men seemed to these women more mysterious and desirable than the men they still cooked for and slept with.

Those who signed up for Grant's courses might have a Scandinavian background or they might have learned something about Norse mythology from Wagner or historical novels. There were also a few who thought he was teaching a Celtic language and for whom everything Celtic had a mystic allure. He spoke to such aspirants fairly roughly from his side of the desk.

"If you want to learn a pretty language go and learn Spanish. Then you can use it if you go to Mexico."

Some took his warning and drifted away. Others seemed to be moved in a personal way by his demanding tone. They worked with a will and brought into his office, into his regulated satisfactory life, the great surprising bloom of their mature female compliance, their tremulous hope of approval.

He chose a woman named Jacqui Adams. She was the opposite of Fiona—short, cushiony, dark-eyed, effusive. A stranger to irony. The affair lasted for a year, until her husband was transferred. When they were saying goodbye in her car, she began to shake uncontrollably. It was as if she had hypothermia. She wrote to him a few times, but he found the tone of her letters overwrought and could not decide how to answer. He let the time for answering slip away while he became magically and unexpectedly involved with a girl who was young enough to be Jacqui's daughter.

For another and more dizzying development had taken place while he was busy with Jacqui. Young girls with long hair and sandalled feet were coming into his office and all but declaring themselves ready for sex. The cautious approaches, the tender intimations of feeling required with Jacqui were out the window. A whirlwind hit him, as it did many others. Scandals burst wide open, with high and painful drama all round but a feeling that somehow it was better so. There were reprisals; there were firings. But those fired went off to teach at smaller, more tolerant colleges or Open Learning

Centers, and many wives left behind got over the shock and took up the costumes, the sexual nonchalance of the girls who had tempted their men. Academic parties, which used to be so predictable, became a minefield. An epidemic had broken out, it was spreading like the Spanish flu. Only this time people ran after contagion, and few between sixteen and sixty seemed willing to be left out.

That was exaggeration, of course. Fiona was quite willing. And Grant himself did not go overboard. What he felt was mainly a gigantic increase in well-being. A tendency to pudginess which he had had since he was twelve years old disappeared. He ran up steps two at a time. He appreciated as never before a pageant of torn clouds and winter sunsets seen from his office window, the charm of antique lamps glowing between his neighbors' living-room curtains, the cries of children in the park, at dusk, unwilling to leave the hill where they'd been tobogganing. Come summer, he learned the names of flowers. In his classroom, after being coached by his nearly voiceless mother-in-law (her affliction was cancer in the throat), he risked reciting the majestic and gory Icelandic ode, the Höfudlausn, composed to honor King Erik Blood-axe by the skald whom that king had condemned to death.

Fiona had never learned Icelandic and she had never shown much respect for the stories that it preserved—the stories that Grant had taught and written about. She referred to their heroes as "old Njal" or "old Snorri." But in the last few years she had developed an interest in the country itself and looked at travel guides. She read about William Morris's trip, and Auden's. She didn't really plan to travel there. She said there ought to be one place you thought about and knew about and maybe longed for but never did get to see.

Nonetheless, the next time he went to Meadowlake, Grant brought Fiona a book he'd found of nineteenth-century watercolors made by a lady traveller to Iceland. It was a Wednesday. He went looking for her at the card tables but didn't see her. A woman called out to him, "She's not here. She's sick."

Her voice sounded self-important and excited—pleased with herself for having recognized him when he knew nothing about her. Perhaps also pleased with all she knew about Fiona, about Fiona's life here, thinking it was maybe more than he knew.

"He's not here, either," she added.

Grant went to find Kristy, who didn't have much time for him. She was talking to a weepy woman who looked like a first-time visitor.

"Nothing really," she said, when he asked what was the matter with Fiona. "She's just having a day in bed today, just a bit of an upset."

Fiona was sitting straight up in the bed. He hadn't noticed, the few times that he had been in this room, that this was a hospital bed and could be cranked up in such a way. She was wearing one of her high-necked maidenly gowns, and her face had a pallor that was like flour paste.

Aubrey was beside her in his wheelchair, pushed as close to the bed as he could get. Instead of the nondescript open-necked shirts he usually wore, he was wearing a jacket and tie. His natty-looking tweed hat was resting on the bed. He looked as if he had been out on important business.

Whatever he'd been doing, he looked worn out by it. He, too, was gray in the face.

They both looked up at Grant with a stony grief-ridden apprehension that turned to relief, if not to welcome, when they saw who he was. Not who they thought he'd be. They were hanging on to each other's hands and they did not let go.

The hat on the bed. The jacket and tie.

It wasn't that Aubrey had been out. It wasn't a question of where he'd been or whom he'd been to see. It was where he was going.

Grant set the book down on the bed beside Fiona's free hand.

"It's about Iceland," he said. "I thought maybe you'd like to look at it."

"Why, thank you," said Fiona. She didn't look at the book.

"Iceland," he said.

She said, "Ice-land." The first syllable managed to hold a tinkle of interest, but the second fell flat. Anyway, it was necessary for her to turn her attention back to Aubrey, who was pulling his great thick hand out of hers.

"What is it?" she said. "What is it, dear heart?"

Grant had never heard her use this flowery expression before.

"Oh all right," she said. "Oh here." And she pulled a handful of tissues from the box beside her bed. Aubrey had begun to weep.

"Here. Here," she said, and he got hold of the Kleenex as well as he could and made a few awkward but lucky swipes at his face. While he was occupied, Fiona turned to Grant.

"Do you by any chance have any influence around here?" she said in a whisper. "I've seen you talking to them. . . ."

Aubrey made a noise of protest or weariness or disgust. Then his upper body pitched forward as if he wanted to throw himself against her. She scrambled half out of bed and caught him and held on to him. It seemed improper for Grant to help her.

"Hush," Fiona was saying. "Oh, honey. Hush. We'll get to see each other. We'll have to. I'll go and see you. You'll come and see me."

Aubrey made the same sound again with his face in her chest and there was nothing Grant could decently do but get out of the room.

"I just wish his wife would hurry up and get here," Kristy said when he ran into her. "I wish she'd get him out of here and cut the agony short.

We've got to start serving supper before long and how are we supposed to get her to swallow anything with him still hanging around?"

Grant said, "Should I stay?"

"What for? She's not sick, you know."

"To keep her company," he said.

Kristy shook her head.

"They have to get over these things on their own. They've got short memories, usually. That's not always so bad."

Grant left without going back to Fiona's room. He noticed that the wind was actually warm and the crows were making an uproar. In the parking lot a woman wearing a tartan pants suit was getting a folded-up wheelchair out of the trunk of her car.

Fiona did not get over her sorrow. She didn't eat at mealtimes, though she pretended to, hiding food in her napkin. She was being given a supplementary drink twice a day—someone stayed and watched while she swallowed it down. She got out of bed and dressed herself, but all she wanted to do then was sit in her room. She wouldn't have had any exercise at all if Kristy, or Grant during visiting hours, hadn't walked her up and down in the corridors or taken her outside. Weeping had left her eyes raw-edged and dim. Her cardigan—if it was hers—would be buttoned crookedly. She had not got to the stage of leaving her hair unbrushed or her nails uncleaned, but that might come soon. Kristy said that her muscles were deteriorating, and that if she didn't improve they would put her on a walker.

"But, you know, once they get a walker they start to depend on it and they never walk much anymore, just get wherever it is they have to go," she said to Grant. "You'll have to work at her harder. Try to encourage her."

But Grant had no luck at that. Fiona seemed to have taken a dislike to him, though she tried to cover it up. Perhaps she was reminded, every time she saw him, of her last minutes with Aubrey, when she had asked him for help and he hadn't helped her.

He didn't see much point in mentioning their marriage now.

The supervisor called him in to her office. She said that Fiona's weight was going down even with the supplement.

"The thing is, I'm sure you know, we don't do any prolonged bed care on the first floor. We do it temporarily if someone isn't feeling well, but if they get too weak to move around and be responsible we have to consider upstairs."

He said he didn't think that Fiona had been in bed that often.

"No. But if she can't keep up her strength she will be. Right now she's borderline."

Grant said that he had thought the second floor was for people whose minds were disturbed.

"That, too," she said.

ॐ

The street Grant found himself driving down was called Blackhawks Lane. The houses all looked to have been built around the same time, perhaps thirty or forty years ago. The street was wide and curving and there were no sidewalks. Friends of Grant and Fiona's had moved to places something like this when they began to have their children, and young families still lived here. There were basketball hoops over garage doors and tricycles in the driveways. Some of the houses had gone downhill. The yards were marked by tire tracks, the windows plastered with tinfoil or hung with faded flags. But a few seemed to have been kept up as well as possible by the people who had moved into them when they were new—people who hadn't had the money or perhaps hadn't felt the need to move on to some place better.

The house that was listed in the phone book as belonging to Aubrey and his wife was one of these. The front walk was paved with flagstones and bordered by hyacinths that stood as stiff as china flowers, alternately pink and blue.

He hadn't remembered anything about Aubrey's wife except the tartan suit he had seen her wearing in the parking lot. The tails of the jacket had flared open as she bent into the trunk of the car. He had got the impression of a trim waist and wide buttocks.

She was not wearing the tartan suit today. Brown belted slacks and a pink sweater. He was right about the waist—the tight belt showed she made a point of it. It might have been better if she didn't, since she bulged out considerably above and below.

She could be ten or twelve years younger than her husband. Her hair was short, curly, artificially reddened. She had blue eyes—a lighter blue than Fiona's—a flat robin's-egg or turquoise blue, slanted by a slight puffiness. And a good many wrinkles, made more noticeable by a walnut-stain makeup. Or perhaps that was her Florida tan.

He said that he didn't quite know how to introduce himself.

"I used to see your husband at Meadowlake. I'm a regular visitor there myself."

"Yes," said Aubrey's wife, with an aggressive movement of her chin.

"How is your husband doing?"

The "doing" was added on at the last moment.

"He's O.K.," she said.

"My wife and he struck up quite a close friendship."

"I heard about that."

"I wanted to talk to you about something if you had a minute."

"My husband did not try to start anything with your wife if that's what you're getting at," she said. "He did not molest her. He isn't capable of it and he wouldn't anyway. From what I heard it was the other way round."

Grant said, "No. That isn't it at all. I didn't come here with any complaints about anything."

"Oh," she said. "Well, I'm sorry. I thought you did. You better come in then. It's blowing cold in through the door. It's not as warm out today as it looks."

So it was something of a victory for him even to get inside.

She took him past the living room, saying, "We'll have to sit in the kitchen, where I can hear Aubrey."

Grant caught sight of two layers of front-window curtains, both blue, one sheer and one silky, a matching blue sofa and a daunting pale carpet, various bright mirrors and ornaments. Fiona had a word for those sort of swooping curtains—she said it like a joke, though the women she'd picked it up from used it seriously. Any room that Fiona fixed up was bare and bright. She would have deplored the crowding of all this fancy stuff into such a small space. From a room off the kitchen—a sort of sunroom, though the blinds were drawn against the afternoon brightness—he could hear the sounds of television.

The answer to Fiona's prayers sat a few feet away, watching what sounded like a ballgame. His wife looked in at him.

She said, "You O.K.?" and partly closed the door.

"You might as well have a cup of coffee," she said to Grant. "My son got him on the sports channel a year ago Christmas. I don't know what we'd do without it."

On the kitchen counters there were all sorts of contrivances and appliances—coffeemaker, food processor, knife sharpener, and some things Grant didn't know the names or uses of. All looked new and expensive, as if they had just been taken out of their wrappings, or were polished daily.

He thought it might be a good idea to admire things. He admired the coffeemaker she was using and said that he and Fiona had always meant to get one. This was absolutely untrue—Fiona had been devoted to a European contraption that made only two cups at a time.

"They gave us that," she said. "Our son and his wife. They live in Kamloops, B.C. They send us more stuff than we can handle. It wouldn't hurt if they would spend the money to come and see us instead."

Grant said philosophically, "I suppose they're busy with their own lives."

"They weren't too busy to go to Hawaii last winter. You could understand it if we had somebody else in the family, closer at hand. But he's the only one."

She poured the coffee into two brown-and-green ceramic mugs that she took from the amputated branches of a ceramic tree trunk that sat on the table.

"People do get lonely," Grant said. He thought he saw his chance now. "If they're deprived of seeing somebody they care about, they do feel sad. Fiona, for instance. My wife."

"I thought you said you went and visited her."

"I do," he said. "That's not it."

Then he took the plunge, going on to make the request he'd come to make. Could she consider taking Aubrey back to Meadowlake, maybe just one day a week, for a visit? It was only a drive of a few miles. Or if she'd like to take the time off—Grant hadn't thought of this before and was rather dismayed to hear himself suggest it—then he himself could take Aubrey out there, he wouldn't mind at all. He was sure he could manage it. While he talked she moved her closed lips and her hidden tongue as if she were trying to identify some dubious flavor. She brought milk for his coffee and a plate of ginger cookies.

"Homemade," she said as she set the plate down. There was challenge rather than hospitality in her tone. She said nothing more until she had sat down, poured milk into her coffee, and stirred it.

Then she said no.

"No. I can't do that. And the reason is, I'm not going to upset him."

"Would it upset him?" Grant said earnestly.

"Yes, it would. It would. That's no way to do. Bringing him home and taking him back. That would just confuse him."

"But wouldn't he understand that it was just a visit? Wouldn't he get into the pattern of it?"

"He understands everything all right." She said this as if he had offered an insult to Aubrey. "But it's still an interruption. And then I've got to get him all ready and get him into the car, and he's a big man, he's not so easy to manage as you might think. I've got to maneuver him into the car and pack his chair and all that and what for? If I go to all that trouble I'd prefer to take him someplace that was more fun."

"But even if I agreed to do it?" Grant said, keeping his tone hopeful and reasonable. "It's true, you shouldn't have the trouble."

"You couldn't," she said flatly. "You don't know him. You couldn't handle him. He wouldn't stand for you doing for him. All that bother and what would he get out of it?"

Grant didn't think he should mention Fiona again.

"It'd make more sense to take him to the mall," she said. "Or now the lake boats are starting to run again, he might get a charge out of going and watching that."

She got up and fetched her cigarettes and lighter from the window above the sink.

"You smoke?" she said.

He said no, thanks, though he didn't know if a cigarette was being offered.

"Did you never? Or did you quit?"

"Quit," he said.

"How long ago was that?"

He thought about it.

"Thirty years. No—more."

He had decided to quit around the time he started up with Jacqui. But he couldn't remember whether he quit first, and thought a big reward was coming to him for quitting, or thought that the time had come to quit, now that he had such a powerful diversion.

"I've quit quitting," she said, lighting up. "Just made a resolution to quit quitting, that's all."

Maybe that was the reason for the wrinkles. Somebody—a woman—had told him that women who smoked developed a special set of fine facial wrinkles. But it could have been from the sun, or just the nature of her skin—her neck was noticeably wrinkled as well. Wrinkled neck, youth-fully full and uptilted breasts. Women of her age usually had these contra-dictions. The bad and good points, the genetic luck or lack of it, all mixed up together. Very few kept their beauty whole, though shadowy, as Fiona had done. And perhaps that wasn't even true. Perhaps he only thought that because he'd known Fiona when she was young. When Aubrey looked at his wife did he see a high-school girl full of scorn and sass, with a tilt to her blue eyes, pursing her fruity lips around a forbidden cigarette?

"So your wife's depressed?" Aubrey's wife said. "What's your wife's name? I forget."

"It's Fiona."

"Fiona. And what's yours? I don't think I was ever told that."

Grant said, "It's Grant."

She stuck her hand out unexpectedly across the table.

"Hello, Grant. I'm Marian."

"So now we know each other's names," she said, "there's no point in not telling you straight out what I think. I don't know if he's still so stuck on seeing your—on seeing Fiona. Or not. I don't ask him and he's not telling me. Maybe just a passing fancy. But I don't feel like taking him back there in case it turns out to be more than that. I can't afford to risk it. I don't want him upset and carrying on. I've got my hands full with him as it is. I don't have any help. It's just me here. I'm it."

"Did you ever consider—I'm sure it's very hard for you—" Grant said. "Did you ever consider his going in there for good?"

He had lowered his voice almost to a whisper but she did not seem to feel a need to lower hers.

"No," she said. "I'm keeping him right here."

Grant said, "Well. That's very good and noble of you." He hoped the word "noble" had not sounded sarcastic. He had not meant it to be.

"You think so?" she said. "Noble is not what I'm thinking about."

"Still. It's not easy."

"No, it isn't. But the way I am, I don't have much choice. I don't have the money to put him in there unless I sell the house. The house is what we own outright. Otherwise I don't have anything in the way of resources. Next year I'll have his pension and my pension, but even so I couldn't afford to keep him there and hang on to the house. And it means a lot to me, my house does."

"It's very nice," said Grant.

"Well, it's all right. I put a lot into it. Fixing it up and keeping it up. I don't want to lose it."

"No. I see your point."

"The company left us high and dry," she said. "I don't know all the ins and outs of it but basically he got shoved out. It ended up with them saying he owed them money and when I tried to find out what was what he just went on saying it's none of my business. What I think is he did something pretty stupid. But I'm not supposed to ask so I shut up. You've been married. You are married. You know how it is. And in the middle of me finding out about this we're supposed to go on this trip and can't get out of it. And on the trip he takes sick from this virus you never heard of and goes into a coma. So that pretty well gets him off the hook."

Grant said, "Bad luck."

"I don't mean he got sick on purpose. It just happened. He's not mad at me anymore and I'm not mad at him. It's just life. You can't beat life."

She flicked her tongue in a cat's businesslike way across her top lip, getting the cookie crumbs. "I sound like I'm quite the philosopher, don't I? They told me out there you used to be a university professor."

"Quite a while ago," Grant said.

"I bet I know what you're thinking," she said. "You're thinking there's a mercenary type of a person."

"I'm not making judgments of that sort. It's your life."

"You bet it is."

He thought they should end on a more neutral note. So he asked her if her husband had worked in a hardware store in the summers, when he was going to school.

"I never heard about it," she said. "I wasn't raised here."

Grant realized he'd failed with Aubrey's wife. Marian. He had thought that what he'd have to contend with would be a woman's natural sexual jealousy—or her resentment, the stubborn remains of sexual jealousy. He had not had any idea of the way she might be looking at things. And yet in some depressing way the conversation had not been unfamiliar to him. That was because it reminded him of conversations he'd had with people in his own family. His relatives, probably even his mother, had thought the way Marian thought. Money first. They had believed that when other people did not think that way it was because they had lost touch with reality. That was how Marian would see him, certainly. A silly person, full of boring knowledge and protected by some fluke from the truth about life. A person who didn't have to worry about holding on to his house and could go around dreaming up the fine generous schemes that he believed would make another person happy. What a jerk, she would be thinking now.

Being up against a person like that made him feel hopeless, exasperated, finally almost desolate. Why? Because he couldn't be sure of holding on to himself, against people like that? Because he was afraid that in the end they were right? Yet he might have married her. Or some girl like that. If he'd stayed back where he belonged. She'd have been appetizing enough. Probably a flirt. The fussy way she had of shifting her buttocks on the kitchen chair, her pursed mouth, a slightly contrived air of menace—that was what was left of the more or less innocent vulgarity of a small-town flirt.

She must have had some hopes when she picked Aubrey. His good looks, his salesman's job, his white-collar expectations. She must have believed that she would end up better off than she was now. And so it often happened with those practical people. In spite of their calculations, their survival instincts, they might not get as far as they had quite reasonably expected. No doubt it seemed unfair.

In the kitchen the first thing he saw was the light blinking on his answering machine. He thought the same thing he always thought now. Fiona. He pressed the button before he took his coat off.

"Hello, Grant. I hope I got the right person. I just thought of something. There is a dance here in town at the Legion supposed to be for singles on Saturday night and I am on the lunch committee, which means I can bring a free guest. So I wondered whether you would happen to be interested in that? Call me back when you get a chance."

A woman's voice gave a local number. Then there was a beep and the same voice started talking again.

"I just realized I'd forgotten to say who it was. Well, you probably recognized the voice. It's Marian. I'm still not so used to these machines. And I wanted to say I realize you're not a single and I don't mean it that way. I'm not either, but it doesn't hurt to get out once in a while. If you are interested you can call me and if you are not you don't need to bother. I just thought you might like the chance to get out. It's Marian speaking. I guess I already said that. O.K. then. Goodbye."

Her voice on the machine was different from the voice he'd heard a short time ago in her house. Just a little different in the first message, more so in the second. A tremor of nerves there, an affected nonchalance, a hurry to get through and a reluctance to let go.

Something had happened to her. But when had it happened? If it had been immediate, she had concealed it very successfully all the time he was with her. More likely it came on her gradually, maybe after he'd gone away. Not necessarily as a blow of attraction. Just the realization that he was a possibility, a man on his own. More or less on his own. A possibility that she might as well try to follow up.

But she'd had the jitters when she made the first move. She had put herself at risk. How much of herself he could not yet tell. Generally a woman's vulnerability increased as time went on, as things progressed. All you could tell at the start was that if there was an edge of it then, there'd be more later. It gave him a satisfaction—why deny it?—to have brought that out in her. To have roused something like a shimmer, a blurring, on the surface of her personality. To have heard in her testy broad vowels this faint plea.

He set out the eggs and mushrooms to make himself an omelette. Then he thought he might as well pour a drink.

Anything was possible. Was that true—was anything possible? For instance, if he wanted to, would he be able to break her down, get her to the point where she might listen to him about taking Aubrey back to Fiona? And not just for visits but for the rest of Aubrey's life. And what would become of him and Marian after he'd delivered Aubrey to Fiona?

Marian would be sitting in her house now, waiting for him to call. Or probably not sitting. Doing things to keep herself busy. She might have fed Aubrey while Grant was buying the mushrooms and driving home. She might now be preparing him for bed. But all the time she would be conscious of the phone, of the silence of the phone. Maybe she would have calculated how long it would take Grant to drive home. His address in the phone book would have given her a rough idea of where he lived. She would calculate how long, then add to that the time it might take him to shop for supper (figuring that a man alone would shop every day). Then a certain amount of time for him to get around to listening to his messages. And as the silence persisted she'd think of other things. Other errands he might have had to do before he got home. Or perhaps a dinner out, a meeting that meant he would not get home at suppertime at all.

What conceit on his part. She was above all things a sensible woman. She would go to bed at her regular time thinking that he didn't look as if he'd be a decent dancer anyway. Too stiff, too professorial.

He stayed near the phone, looking at magazines, but he didn't pick it up when it rang again.

"Grant. This is Marian. I was down in the basement putting the wash in the dryer and I heard the phone and when I got upstairs whoever it was had hung up. So I just thought I ought to say I was here. If it was you and if you are even home. Because I don't have a machine, obviously, so you couldn't leave a message. So I just wanted. To let you know." The time was now twenty-five after ten.

"Bye."

He would say that he'd just got home. There was no point in bringing to her mind the picture of his sitting here weighing the pros and cons.

Drapes. That would be her word for the blue curtains—drapes. And why not? He thought of the ginger cookies so perfectly round that she had to announce they were homemade, the ceramic coffee mugs on their ceramic tree, a plastic runner, he was sure, protecting the hall carpet. A high-gloss exactness and practicality that his mother had never achieved but would have admired—was that why he could feel this twinge of bizarre and unreliable affection? Or was it because he'd had two more drinks after the first?

The walnut-stain tan—he believed now that it was a tan—of her face and neck would most likely continue into her cleavage, which would be deep, crêpey-skinned, odorous and hot. He had that to think of as he dialled the number that he had already written down. That and the practical sensuality of her cat's tongue. Her gemstone eyes.

Fiona was in her room but not in bed. She was sitting by the open window, wearing a seasonable but oddly short and bright dress. Through the window came a heady warm blast of lilacs in bloom and the spring manure spread over the fields.

She had a book open in her lap.

She said, "Look at this beautiful book I found. It's about Iceland. You wouldn't think they'd leave valuable books lying around in the rooms. But I think they've got the clothes mixed up—I never wear yellow."

"Fiona," he said.

"Are we all checked out now?" she said. He thought the brightness of her voice was wavering a little. "You've been gone a long time."

"Fiona, I've brought a surprise for you. Do you remember Aubrey?"

She stared at Grant for a moment, as if waves of wind had come beating into her face. Into her face, into her head, pulling everything to rags. All rags and loose threads.

"Names elude me," she said harshly.

Then the look passed away as she retrieved, with an effort, some bantering grace. She set the book down carefully and stood up and lifted her arms to put them around him. Her skin or her breath gave off a faint new smell, a smell that seemed to Grant like green stems in rank water.

"I'm happy to see you," she said, both sweetly and formally. She pinched his earlobes, hard.

"You could have just driven away," she said. "Just driven away without a care in the world and forsook me. Forsooken me. Forsaken."

He kept his face against her white hair, her pink scalp, her sweetly shaped skull.

He said, "Not a chance."

18

Thoreau's Laundry

❧ *Ann Harleman*

The morning's first client—she never called them patients—appeared on the list as Junius Johns. This was followed by the usual basics: M, 8, left ear, AA. Sex, age, presenting problem, origin (auto accident). In the margin a penciled notation from Edwin, her receptionist, read: "Mad Mom+ Relatives."

Celia put her elbows on the desk and let her forehead sink onto her palms. She was tired. Not just tired—weary. Simon's catheter had gone AWOL at one in the morning, and they'd spent the rest of the night in the ER. (How many nights did that make, now? How many hours?) Noise and cold and too-bright lights and too-bright student doctors. Repeating her husband's history, over and over, to a succession of twelve-year-olds in lab coats and stethoscopes. Her husband in pain, and nothing in the world she could do about it. By the time Doctor Mikhailov entered the cubicle and took Simon's hand between both of his, the sun was up. A cautious November sun that barely reddened the sky above the parking lot, where the cold fell like a blessing on Celia's hospital-hot face and winter birds measured out early-morning sounds in the trees overhead. She called Leslie on her cell phone and asked her to meet Simon's ambulance at the house when they'd finished with him ("No prob!" That was Leslie, best friend ever, and Celia's cousin to boot. "I'll call you and let you know he's okay, okay?") Then she drove straight to the office, where wonderful Edwin had had a cappuccino and croissant waiting.

Celia brushed the silky crumbs off her desk and opened the drawer where she kept an assortment of puppets for child clients. Though usually the adults needed the distraction more. To Celia's continuing surprise, people found what she did for a living grisly. Maxillofacial prosthetist: that was the official name, the phrase her accountant put at the top of each page of her income tax return. She made eyes and ears and noses—and any other

---

parts of a face that might be needed—for people who were missing them. People whom cancer or fire or gunshot had ravaged. People whom the plastic surgeons had given up on.

She took out the first puppet she touched and pulled it on over her left hand, wriggling her thumb and little finger into the arms, comforted by the feel of velvet. An ancient, bearded little man in a midnight-blue gown scattered with gold stars, and a pointed magician's cap. When she crooked her index finger, he nodded. She buzzed Edwin, two shorts: *Ready*.

The door opened. A gaggle of female voices. Then a wheelchair appeared—really a sort of wheeled chaise lounge, containing a small black boy with both legs outstretched—flanked by three large women in flowing flowered smocks, all talking at once.

"—you *know* he never—"

"I'm just sayin'—"

"—that's what *anybody* gotta—"

Behind this procession Edwin hovered, rolling his eyes. Celia put up her hands and shouted, "Stop!"

Instant silence, followed, inexplicably, by giggles. The largest of the three women, standing beside the wheelchair in magenta silk, put a hand across her mouth.

"You must be Junius," Celia said to the boy. "I'm Celia."

The boy's eyes, large and liquid, met hers for a heartbeat, then shifted to the puppet. His left leg wore a cast from hip to ankle; the right was bare, except for a layer of what looked like raw chopped meat spread all along his thigh. The harvest site for a skin graft, Celia knew. The surgeon who'd referred Junius believed in old-fashioned gauze dressings soaked in iodoform.

He don't talk hardly at all, doctor," the woman in magenta said. "Since the accident."

"I'm not a doc—"

"Barely a peep!" cried one of the other women, and the third chimed in, "Lord knows!"

Edwin brought two more chairs from the outer office, and the women sat down in a flurry of silk, Magenta beside the wheelchair, Carnation and Tiger Lily behind it. Edwin cocked his head, and his eyebrows (so black and perfect that she'd always wondered if he penciled them) rose. This was as far as he went with worrying about her, which was why she'd looked for a male secretary in the first place. There were too many concerned females in her life already. Celia mouthed *Thanks*, and he left, closing the door behind him.

Celia turned to Magenta. "Mrs. Johns? I understand you're—"

The woman leaned forward. "The hospital made us come here," she said, spitting the words. Edwin had been right, as usual: this woman was mad.

"The *insurance* made us. No more surgery—that's what they say. My boy don't show promise. He ain't a *candidate.*"

"Whatever *that* means," Carnation said, and Tiger Lily added, "Lord knows!"

Celia sighed. This Greek chorus was going to get old fast. The length of Junius's wheelchair put the whole group at a slightly theatrical distance from her desk. Junius himself sat chewing gum with downcast eyes. When his jaw moved, the hole where his left ear should have been pulsed faintly. She was always surprised at how small the aural opening actually was.

She rose and went around the desk and crouched down next to him, on his left side. He didn't look up. She raised the puppet in front of his face and bent her thumb to make it bow. "I'm Merlin!" she said, in a deep, plummy voice. "I make magic."

The boy's mouth twitched. He raised his head, but he didn't look at Celia, only at the puppet.

"Can't see what good playin' dolls gonna do. Or false ears, either. The Lord alone can help my boy now."

"Lord help him!"

"Yeah, Lord!"

Celia turned her head and shot the three women a look—what Simon called her dark-blue look—useful in ER waiting rooms. There was a subsiding rustle of silk around three sets of knees. Then, silence.

Inches now from Junius's head, she had a good view. Stumpy petals of flesh ringed the aural opening, where the lobe and helix had been sheared away; only the tragus remained. A webbing of scar tissue made the skin look like hammered bronze. It wasn't ugly; it just didn't look like an ear. She saw exactly where Doctor Prout would implant the gold-and-titanium abutments her silicone ear would snap onto. (She wouldn't mention that now; better to leave breaking the news about more surgery to the surgeon.) Junius had stopped chewing gum, and she could feel him trembling. His hand gripped her wrist.

"Ho!" she said, in Merlin's voice. "You look like a fine, strong lad. A good candidate for magic."

She felt the boy stiffen.

"We don't believe in magic," his mother said. "We believe in Jesus."

Celia looked up. The woman smiled, not apologetically but as if to say, *You'll never understand, so don't even try.* A feeling Celia knew well.

Junius said nothing.

Celia rose and went around to the boy's right to look at his good ear. The one she would make for him had to match this one, imperfections and all. She noted the wrinkle where the lobe attached, the too- sharply folded helix that gave the top a Spock-like point. Black skin was harder to match than white: she'd start with umber and burnt sienna, maybe add a little monastral red.

She felt the boy's breath, with its smell of spearmint, graze her cheek. She thought, This at least is something I can do.

The evening air was full of unshed rain. In the thickening darkness a sea-smelling wind stirred the few leaves left on the trees. Homeward, she drove more slowly than she needed to. Headlights loomed suddenly behind her, slewed sideways, shot past, loomed again.

Simon would be waiting for her in the ground-floor sunporch-turned-sickroom. Would this be a good night, or a bad?

Low, womanly hills replaced the clustered lights of the city. Celia turned the heat up. At the junction where 101 split off from Route 6 she looked for the turkey that lived on the triangle of grass there, in the glow of the floodlighted sign announcing the Township of Jerimoth. For the last few years there'd been an overabundance of turkeys in rural areas. She peered through the smoky blue twilight. *If it paces past, Simon won't be mean. If it turns its head toward me, he will.*

Multiple sclerosis had made their marriage a ménage a trois. It was as simple, as complicated, as that.

"You have lucky eyes and a high heart."

The first thing Simon ever said to her, that June night eighteen years ago. (My Shakespeare professor, her cousin Leslie had said, dragging Celia the length of the lantern-lit veranda, their long taffeta skirts rustling. He's totally gorgeous, you've *got* to meet him.) Behind them the orchestra began tuning up, quick interrogative sounds.

"Dance with me. Every dance. With me."

Impossibly romantic; but then, they'd been impossibly romantic. Impossibly young (her). Impossibly married (him). So impossible that they had to happen.

Her key stuttered in the lock, reluctance made physical. There was the breath-held moment—every night, now—What will I find? (Husband on the floor, blood pooling under his temple; husband sprawled headfirst down the steps to the basement; husband slumped sideways in his wheelchair, raising a book upside-down in his good hand to shelter tears of fury.) She forced the key all the way in, pushed open the heavy oak door.

"Seal? That . . . you?"

His words were halting but clear, his voice strong enough to carry across the living room. Celia's breath escaped through dry lips. Relieved, she bent to pick up the mail from the floor below the mail slot. Electric bill, gas bill, various catalogues, a flyer from the MS Society's Well Spouse Group.

Simon looked up as she paused in the archway between the living room and the sunporch. For an instant his face wore the expression she remembered from years ago—from all those meetings-after-long-absence, in those first years before they'd been able to marry—*I'm so glad to see you.*

The tip of his tongue touched his mustache, then retreated. "How was . . . your day?"

His eyes crinkled at the corners with the old wryness. Simon's sense of the absurd was the thing, besides sex, that had made her fall for him in the (impossible) first place.

Relief brought the itch of tears to her throat. She swallowed. "Fine. How was yours? What's new?"

"New York. New . . . Jersey."

"New . . . Mexico," they said, in unison.

Eighteen years together, eight of them healthy: Professor Simon Feldstein had taught her a few things. Some Yiddish words, how to make risotto, quite a few lines from Shakespeare, and a way of joking that kept you from falling off the edge of the world. Celia kissed him lightly on the mustache, threw her parka over a chair, handed him the remote. The sound of the Weather Channel followed her into the kitchen.

A good night, then. In a way, the bad nights were easier. The good nights made her remember. The good nights disarmed her.

And, yes, you ARE above the freezing mark, Providence, but it sure doesn't FEEL like that!

Celia opened the freezer and peered inside. The phone rang.

When she picked up, her mother's voice demanded, "Where were you?"

"God, Mom—I'm sorry. I forgot all about lunch. Something came up. An emergency."

"Simon? What happened? Is he—"

"Not Simon." Celia took out a frozen dinner and let the freezer door slam shut on her lie. "A client."

"Because if it was Simon—"

"Mom! Simon's okay—he's fine. So, what did you do this afternoon? Teeth?" Her mother's current lover, whom Leslie had christened the Priapodontist, was in the middle of replacing her entire lifetime accumulation of fillings with gold.

"Nothing. After lunch you and I were supposed to go shopping." (And how she loved it, Celia thought: The cries of What?-You're-her *mother?*

Bridling and beaming.) "You know, you'd look slimmer in one of those new trumpet skirts. Maybe with a cropped sweater."

"I've got to go, Mom. Time for Simon's meds. I'll call you later."

She put her dinner in the oven, "Hungry Man" servings of fried chicken and mashed potatoes and corn frozen in their own neatly partitioned tinfoil tray, a depraved appetite she'd recently developed. Then she began to grind the evening meds with a mortar and pestle.

From the day Simon had been diagnosed, almost eleven years ago, her mother had made no secret of what she thought would be best for every-one concerned. Simon in a nursing home; Celia with, married or not, a real mate; Bess herself beamingly promoted, at long last, to What?-You're-a-*grandmother?*-hood. It terrified Celia that her mother's vision matched the one (the impossible one) that tattooed itself across her closed eyelids every night as she lay awake in the bed next to Simon's.

The medications, mingling and dissolving, smelled like sulfur. When the powder was as fine as she could get it, she stirred it into a beaker of warm water until it dissolved in a pastel cloud.

Colder air means BLACK ICE! We'll have an update on that later tonight.

In the sunporch she turned off Simon's feeding pump and detached it from the G-tube inserted in her husband's stomach, slowly poured the meds solution into the G-tube, then hung a fresh bag of liquid diet on his IV pole and hooked it up to the pump. "Chief . . . nourisher . . . in life's feast," Simon murmured in his Shakespeare voice. Celia reattached the feeding tube to the G-tube. Snapping them together, she pulled too hard on the end that protruded from the pale, freckled flesh of Simon's belly, and heard his sharp, in-drawn breath. "Sorry!" she said.

He shook his head. "It's . . . okay."

She rose and turned the pump back on, stood listening for its slow, meditative clicks.

In the little bathroom she assembled the paraphernalia for his shot. Somehow, no matter how careful she was with things—G-tube, catheter, hypodermic—she always hurt him. The other Well Spouses in her support group never hurt their partners.

Kneeling beside Simon's wheelchair, she breathed in his familiar smell: baby powder, urine, and something less definable, the remote, forest odor of decay. Okay. Choose today's spot (there was a complicated rotation sys-tem involving arms, thighs, and belly), swab spot, insert fresh needle into holder, suck in sterile water 1.3 milliliters, inject water into ampule, turn ampule upside down until contents mix with water, suck in contents 1.3 milliliters (no air bubbles! flick with fingernail to disperse), hold needle poised in one hand, pinch husband's flesh between thumb and forefinger of other. People assumed Celia would be deft. Useless to protest that, even counting her prosthesis training from the VA a dozen years ago, she'd gone to art school, not med school. People didn't see the difference between handling something inert and handling something that breathed.

Our Little Marvel Snowblower does all this, and MORE!

Simon kept his eyes on the TV screen. The needle glittered in the lamplight. She plunged it in. He winced.

Celia let her breath out. That was it, until bedtime. She thought of these routines, collectively, as a sort of quilting stitch that held their pieced-together life in place. She didn't know how Simon viewed them.

Hug him, at least touch him. Give him his body back. Slowly she drew the palm of her hand across his neck, under his woolen shirt. The skin felt warm and grainy. His eyes closed in pleasure like a cat's. She gathered up her medical paraphernalia. In the bathroom she threw the used needle into the big red rubber Sharps container that squatted in one corner. The skull-and-crossbones on its belly leered at her.

At last she sat down next to Simon's wheelchair with Hungry Man on her lap and a glass of white Zinfandel on the table beside her. Two years ago, when the G-tube was inserted permanently into Simon's stomach, they'd agreed—or rather, Simon, with the generosity she remembered from the Well Years, had insisted—that they would still eat together. Now he watched her, and she let him: a gustatory voyeur.

His nose twitched. Wistfully?

"It tastes terrible," she assured him. "It tastes like . . . like breaded toilet paper and shoe buttons," and was rewarded with his brief bark of a laugh.

That's it for you folks in New England. Stay tuned for STORM STORIES!

Simon's good hand fumbled across the remote until it met the "Off" button. Silence. He said, "Cheers!"

She raised her glass in a toast to his IV pole and drank deeply, the wine stinging her throat. Then she told him about her day.

Bedtime was hoisting Simon up, coaxing the flesh together; was the weight of him, wheelchair to grab bars to commode to bed, thudding onto her shoulders and traveling down her spine; was the separate sigh from each of them when at last he lay, more or less straight, in the bed; was the cool gust from the down quilt as it settled over him; was the snap of the bedside light, extinguished.

Like putting a child to bed—the child they hadn't had. Plenty of time, they used to think.

Simon fell asleep quickly, the way he always did. Downstairs, Celia poured another glass of wine and settled into the sofa, settled into the part of the day that was hers, and thought about her lover.

Max.

Was it only a week ago they were hiking in Maine? Three hundred feet above the Atlantic, in a light snow, the path wound up and up between stony banks and pine trees, slippery and steep. When they came out, finally, onto the view of the shining little harbor at Rogue Bluff, it took her breath away. Her breath—not theirs. Max, who for the last half-hour had been a good twenty yards ahead, didn't stop to wait for her. To see this together: the sheer drop to the sea, the curve of the bay, the blue-green water with its flock of boats sheltering beneath the cliff. Where the path—rough stone steps now, winding down and down into the trees—continued, Max's square Scandinavian head and shoulders disappeared around a bend.

The following day, when she woke up, he was gone. Above her head the skylight in the conical cloth roof of the yurt showed a rose-colored sky. Sunrise. Warmth and light and emptiness. The woodstove glowed red; he'd stoked the fire. On the rough plank floor beside her sleeping bag he'd left a note.

Celia's cousin Leslie was the only person in her life who knew about Max. She'd met him in the spring, a few weeks after he and Celia had become lovers. The Contender, Leslie had christened him. He was the first one she'd ever liked. She had nicknames for all of Celia's lovers over the last decade: the Flake, the Field Marshal, Mr. Something-for-Nothing, the Thief of Joy. ("You said it, not me," Leslie told her when she protested this last one. "You said he ruined every good time.") Yet who, Celia wondered, could blame these men for not being able to handle what the Field Marshal used to call "the spouse issue"?

Leslie was the one who, whenever Celia got depressed about all this—whenever, over the past ten years, she'd referred to herself as the Well Slut—said, *No.*

"You're trying to make a life out of the pieces you have, Seal. That's all anybody ever does. It's just, your pieces are harder to fit together than most."

The afternoon's first call was her mother. Celia wedged the phone between her ear and her shoulder and looked over the appointment schedule Edwin had just laid on her desk. "Read any good books lately?" she said into the phone. Bess read two or three at a time, putting one down and picking up another, the way a chain smoker smoked.

"At the moment I'm reading the biography of Thoreau Leslie gave me for my birthday. And I'm in the middle of that fantastic new book, *Geyser Life*. Don't change the subject. Are you gaining weight?"

"*Guys Are Life?* I don't *think* so."

"No, no. *Geyser Life*. Old Faithful, and all that. Great photographs. You could do worse, Cecilia."

"Worse photographs?"

"Worse than give men a place in your life."

If you only knew, Celia thought. So many men; so little place.

"It wouldn't hurt Simon. He'd never know."

He *doesn't* know. And he never will. No one but Leslie will ever know about Max, or any of the others.

"You'd get out more. No wonder you're gaining weight. Thoreau said, 'Live the life you've imagined.' He said, 'Go confidently in the direction of your dreams.' Where do you ever go in the evenings, besides Well Spouse meetings?"

"We've been through this a hundred times. Listen, I can't talk right now. My one-thirty is out in the waiting room. The little boy, remember, the one who got hit by—"

"Cecilia—"

"Gotta go, Mom. Love you. Bye."

Celia's studio occupied half of the top floor of an old factory building in Pawtucket. Cold clear light poured in through the tall windows. The big, high-ceilinged room held the welcoming smells of plaster, paint, linseed oil. She turned on both space heaters, then took off her jacket and hung it on a peg by the door. The boom-box, tuned to an oldies station, drowned out the rap music from the painter's studio next door. A group Celia's mother had loved when Celia was in grade school sang about how hard life used to be. As always when she was in the studio, her spirits rose. Home ground: here she was deft, decisive, sure.

The mold for Mrs. de Carvalho had cured. Celia took a tiny jeweler's hammer from the tool rack above her worktable and began to tap the plaster around the edges. One of the first prostheses Celia had ever made, Mrs. de Carvalho's silicone eye—its pale green iris dusty with age, like the bloom on a grape—had had to be remade twice over the last twelve years, to keep pace with its aging mate.

She worked on the lashes most of the afternoon. It was a job requiring laser-like concentration, which Celia liked because of the peace it brought her. Nothing stilled obsessive rumination like the need to lift minute hairs, two or three at a time, in tiny tweezers the size of a needle, and punch them into the silicone eyelid at precisely the right angle, over and over. On the wall at the back of the worktable was a mirror about a foot wide, to which she held up the eye from time to time to get a fresh view. She worked until the eye, checked against photos of Mrs. de Carvalho's real one, had almost all the imperfections of its mate. The cornea and iris were excellent matches, but the sclera—she hadn't been able to get the precise mottling of yellow on white. She sighed. As if in commiseration, the radio began to play "I Can't Get No Satisfaction." Celia blew a few stray lash hairs off the eye, so lifelike she almost waited for it to blink, then put it into a gray plastic case and set it on the Outgoing Shelf. Perfect is the Enemy of Good—that was what they'd taught at the VA. In the end you didn't so much finish a piece as abandon it.

The studio's many-paned windows gleamed with sunset. Feeling she'd earned a break, Celia took the cardboard box marked "JOHNS, J. 11/04" from the Pending Shelf. Junius's mother had cancelled his initial fitting yesterday, without explanation. Celia's disappointment had, she knew, been out of scale, almost to the point of tears. She'd made Edwin—eyebrows raised at the inappropriateness—phone Junius's house. There'd been no answer.

She wiped the surface of her worktable with a chamois, sweeping silicone fragments and dust and hairs onto the floor. Then she opened the box and lifted the two wax models—Junius's remaining ear and *her* ear—from their nest of gray silk. The replacement ear went on a stand in front of the mirror; the other one, next to it. She began—quite unnecessarily, since she'd finished carving it on Tuesday—comparing the mirrored ear with the other one. That little fold at the top of the helix. The angle was off about ten degrees. Of its own accord her hand reached for a small wax knife.

Why hadn't they shown up for the fitting? The impression taking last week had gone all right, a stoic Junius not even complaining, as most kids did, about the smell of the alginate or the creepy feel of it pouring over his skin. Eyes on the mirrored ear, Celia shaved minute curls of wax from the top, making it more Spock-like. Junius was one of her pro bono patients, referred by the children's unit at Shriners Burn Institute in Boston. A lot of people didn't like taking charity; maybe his redoubtable mama was one of them. When he finally did come in for the initial fitting, he'd be disappointed, of course. They all were, at first. It was too hard to imagine, when she held the colorless wax pretend ear to the ravaged opening, the lifelike eventual ear that would be there. Celia sometimes thought the most exhausting part of her work was the *convincing*. She had to do the imagining for both of them.

She was so absorbed that when her cell phone vibrated against her stomach—the strange not-quite-tickling sensation she always thought must be like feeling your unborn baby move—she jumped and dropped the wax knife. Her cell phone number was reserved for emergencies only. She took it out of her pocket and punched the "On" button.

Simon lay on the gurney under a stiff hospital sheet that left his feet bare. Corrugated plastic tubing, like a pastel vacuum-cleaner hose, protruded from his mouth and snaked its way to a monitor on a stand. Celia stood at Simon's head, the edge of the gurney pressing into her pelvis, and looked down. The ventilator's clear plastic mask flattened his beard and mustache; his face was alarmingly pale. As if in response to the sheer force of her attention, his eyelids began to flutter. *Open!* she said silently. But they didn't.

After some minutes, she pulled the stiff sheet over his feet, which, as her hand brushed them, felt like stone. Then she settled into the slippery vinyl visitor's chair to wait for Doctor Mikhailov. Folding her arms for warmth—why were hospitals always so cold?—she closed her eyes and let her ears fill with the rhythmic suck and sigh of the ventilator. When she opened them again, Simon's head was turned toward her and he was looking at her, his lips—or was it just the pressure of the plastic mask?—curved in the beginnings of a smile.

"*You* have got a *lovely* butt!"

Through the door, flung back so energetically it bounced off the bookcase next to it, came Junius in his chair. His mother, who was pushing it, was speaking over her shoulder to Edwin.

Relief—here they were, though without an appointment—flooded Celia. "Sit down, please," she said.

Edwin hovered. She'd never seen him blush before. She waved him away, and the door closed behind him. Mama parked the wheelchair alongside Celia's desk and settled her voluminous skirts—saffron silk, this time—into the visitor's chair. Her face beneath the broad brim of a fake leopard-skin hat wore a bright, expectant look. Maybe she'd mixed up the appointment times?

"I'm so sorry," Celia said. "I don't have the model—the ear—here in the office. We weren't expecting you. Can you come back tomorrow? Edwin will tell you what time." To Junius, she added, "I think you'll like it. It's going to look totally real."

Junius turned his head away and looked out the window.

"Junius! I don't know what's got into him, Doctor. Why, when we got on the bus he was so excited!"

Celia tried again. "You'll be able to put it on and take it off by yourself. Just snap and unsnap."

Without turning his head, Junius shrugged.

"It's very cool. Your buddies will be impressed."

Junius removed his gaze from the window and said, "He didn't stop. I'm gettin' down from the school bus, and I see this car coming, this blue van, and I see the driver lookin' at me, through the windshield. I *see* him."

"Simon'll be discharged soon," Leslie said.

They sat, Celia and Leslie, bundled in sweaters with quilts over their knees, in Leslie's dying garden. Joe had taken their son, Tommy, up to Boston, to the Museum of Science, where a special exhibit featured two hundred species of frogs, most of them deadly. The late morning sun was bright but cold. It gave Leslie's hair a dark crow's-wing shine. Leaves, faded to rose and ochre and brown, littered the flagstones and lay in drifts along the high cedar fence, and the nearly leafless maples threw an intricate net of shadows over the two women.

"You've been talking to my mother."

"Aunt Bess has nothing to do with it." Leslie's high-backed wooden chair creaked as she moved. She was incapable of talking without gestures. "But she did happen to mention that Simon's doctor thinks this time, when he leaves the ICU, he should go somewhere with round-the-clock care. Round-the-clock *nurses*. A nursing home, Seal."

She couldn't afford to get mad at Leslie. Without Leslie, she'd go under. "In the first place, I can take care of him. I *do* take care of him. In the second place, he'd never go."

"You're at work all day. He falls. Concussions, a hematoma, stitches. All those trips to the ER. He's the most pigheaded man I know. One of these days when he thinks he can manage—when he thinks, 'What am I, Professor Simon Feldstein, doing in a fucking wheelchair?'—he'll stand up and take off across the living room and break a hip. Then where'll you be? Where'll *he* be?"

Celia couldn't deny that it was a relief to drive homeward each evening in the deepening dusk with her husband in safe hands, no one waiting for her at the end of her journey. She picked up one of Tommy's action figures, which lay in a heap on the low wooden table between her and Leslie, and began bending its arms and legs into impossible positions. Always before, she'd been able to count on Leslie to understand that she couldn't send Simon away, not for his sake but for her own. That his presence, however diminished, was as necessary to her as breathing. Losing him, she would lose herself, Celia, the person she'd been all her adult life.

Leslie waved a hand. "If he insists on coming home, you could get East Bay Nursing to send somebody. They're good. We had them when Dad died. Then you could go up to Rogue Bluff and stay in the yurt. Get your bearings. Commute down here to your office a couple of days a week, or move the whole enchilada up there. I'll bet the VA and Shriners'd come to *you*. You're the best around."

Not so much best, as only. Most maxillofacial prosthetists went where the money was: either Hollywood or the CIA. Celia rolled the action figure between her palms. He was a superhero, she could tell from the cape and tights.

"Seal! Are you listening? Say Simon does insist on coming home. If you move out, he'll have to face how much he demands from you. How much help he needs now, to survive."

Celia thought, I should never have let her read Max's letter. Then she wouldn't know he offered me the yurt.

"Leslie—for God's sake! I couldn't just move out. You know I couldn't."

Leslie went on as if Celia hadn't spoken. "How many times have you told me, Maine lets you breathe. And Simon will be safe."

"Safety isn't the point. No one lives in order to be *safe*."

Leslie gathered up the manuscript pages she'd been working on when Celia arrived—she translated from Spanish and Portuguese, mostly legal and business documents, into English—and Tommy's Game Boy and assorted superheroes. "Let's go in. We can have tea. Peppermint, almond, or licorice? And there's some of Joe's *panettone*."

If even Leslie thought she should let go of Simon, then Celia had no allies at all. Despair washed through her. Her eyes moved over the wild, leaf-strewn margins of the garden, the yellowed stalks of what used to be snapdragons, the tall skeletons of hollyhocks and sunflowers. The sun was directly overhead now—it was almost noon—but she felt as cold as when they'd first sat down. "Fear no more the heat o' the sun," she murmured.

"What?"

"Shakespeare. It was the first thing Simon said when they took him off the ventilator yesterday. At least, it sounded like that was what he said."

Leslie rose, sloughing leaves off her lap. "Like some unknown nobody said: You can't prevent the birds of sorrow from flying over your head, but you can keep them from building a nest in your hair."

On warm nights Max liked to open the plastic skylight at the top of the yurt. Moonlight seemed to enter their bodies. The fragrance of the pines mingled with the smell of her own sweat and then with the scent they made together; the ringing of the crickets mixed with her own quick cries.

Afterwards, she lay with Max's body folded around hers and the sleeping bag folded around them both. Sometimes he snored, very lightly, a matter-of-fact sound, beautiful and ordinary. Sometimes the last thing she heard was the swift whisper of the zipper as he zipped them in, like the sound of a bird taking flight.

"I'll call you back this afternoon, Mom."

"What was it Simon used to say? When we die, God will reproach us for all the beauty He put on earth that we declined to enjoy."

"I've got a full waiting room out there. Simon never said any such thing."

"Thoreau, then. People need partners, Seal. We're mammals, after all."

"Drop it, Ma."

"If you fell in love, you'd feel better. All those endorphins. And don't call me Ma. You know perfectly well that no one would take me for your mother."

It had been August when he told her. More than eight years ago, now. For a week they'd been waiting, disbelief buttressing defiance, for the results of the MRI. It was a hot, somber, dark-skied afternoon. It was—though she didn't realize this until years later—the very last time his illness was the same experience for both of them. She bit her lip hard, blood salty on her tongue, so as not to cry. They made love, not desperately (that would come later), not despairingly (that would come later still), but determinedly. Like two people trying to say everything—past, future, *now*—in a single telegram.

Afterwards, they lay with their cooling bodies tight together, their heads on the same pillow. She turned her face away so that he wouldn't taste her tears. Her hair, long then, tugged painfully against her scalp where his head held it fast to the pillow. A hot breeze sifted through the open window, and they could hear the far-off rumbling of a slowly approaching thunderstorm.

"Everything that grows," he'd whispered into her hair, in his Shakespeare voice, "holds in perfection but a little moment."

"A yurt—that's some kind of tent, right? Are you crazy?"

"You've been talking to Leslie. That's *her* idea. It's just an idea."

"All alone in the *woods?*"

"Mom. I have to hang up now. I haven't seen Simon yet today."

"You could stay here, in the spare room. Even Thoreau went home once a week. Did you know that? He took his laundry home to his mother."

Celia settled in her chair and looked down at the day's roster. Henry Threadgill, referred from Shriners Burn Institute—M, 74, B—for the third time this year ("Nose itch—a bitch," Edwin had written next to his name); Amar Singh, the beautiful young man from Bombay, whose dark-blue turban hid the ear misshapen since birth; Mrs. de Carvalho. But where was Junius? Celia's stomach gave a little leap, anticipating the moment when she would snap his new car into place. Anticipating the sight of his face looking sideways into the mirror she'd hold up to him.

She buzzed Edwin.

The intercom crackled. "Yeah?"

"Junius Johns. He's coming back today for his fitting. What time?"

"They cancelled. There was a message from big mama on the voicemail this morning. I put old Threadgill in their spot."

Relax. Breathe.

Celia undid the waistband button on her good gray pants, breathed deeper, and looked out the window, blinking back tears. Outside, it was a perfect day. Burning blue sky; the last deep-red leaves twirling down from the Japanese apple, released; the sun coming in at a golden slant through its polished branches.

What was it the nuns had taught them, in Saturday catechism class? They'd had to chant it, a dozen seven-year-old voices piping in unison, hands clapping the beat. The SINS against HOPE are PreSUMPtion and DESPAIR. Why would Junius blow her off? They'd had a rapport. He'd spoken. Even his mother had been amazed. Why would she not bring him back?

But maybe that *was* why. That's what Simon would say. The Theory of Paradoxical Causality, he used to call it. The very reason people should do something was often the reason they didn't.

The thing was, she could not imagine it: the hopeful sound of zippers, the shuffle of luggage down the ramp into the driveway, the wheelchair in the doorway jerking around, presenting her with Simon's eloquent back. Couldn't imagine looking, one day not long from now, out her office window at her loaded pickup, its blue tarp dusted with the season's first snow. Couldn't imagine driving, at the end of the afternoon's work, not west, but north.

19

The Yawn

❧ Rachel Hadas

My visiting tall son
is sleepy. His sweet gape
brings back his father's yawn.
Seeing our lost husband and lost father
suddenly conjured up, I laugh. My son
frowns. Does he think
it's at him I'm laughing?
The cat opens her mouth to mew.
The orphaned piano: it yawns, too.

Mrs. Dumpty

❧ Chana Bloch

The last time the doctors gave up
I put the pieces together
and bought him a blue wool jacket, a shirt
and a tie with scribbles of magenta,
brown buckle shoes. I dressed him
and sat him down
with a hankie in his pocket folded into points.
Then a shell knit slowly
over his sad starched heart.

He'd laugh and dangle his long legs and call out,
What a fall that was!
And I'd sing the refrain,
What a fall!

And now he's at my door again, begging
in that leaky voice,
and I start wiping the smear
from his broken face.

Chana Bloch, "Mrs. Dumpty" and "Visiting Hours Are Over," from *Mrs. Dumpty*. Winner of the 1998 Felix Pollak Prize in Poetry. Copyright © 1998 by the Board of Regents of the University of Wisconsin System. Reprinted by permission of The University of Wisconsin Press.

21

Visiting Hours Are Over

❧ Chana Bloch

Down the hall past the half-
closed doors
a body
crumpled on every bed
striped pajamas three pills
in a pleated cup past the windows
double-glazed against
the cold past the waxy
sansevieria past the lead apron
of hospital drapes
down the front steps into rain
two blocks
to the car
I run
just to feel
my feet
slap the
pavement my hands
slam against my sides
cold wet
cold slippery wet
I don't
open the umbrella

He Read to Her

& *Anne Brashler*

She locked the bathroom door, sprayed the small closed room with lemon odor, then removed her robe. The colostomy bag was full and leaking; brown stains seeped down her belly and across old scars, new scars, old stretch marks. Her stomach looked like a map of dirt roads. "Crap," she said. She cupped her hand under the bag, holding it like a third breast, then held her breath long enough to break the seal, remove the bag, and quickly tie its contents into a white plastic container. Her colostomy resembled a brown puckered rose.

The bathroom filled with billowy steam as she stayed under the shower. When her husband rapped on the door, she said, "I'm fine. Leave me alone." As she stepped from the tub, refreshed and clean, the puckered rose exploded with bile, shooting brown stinking liquid over the sink, the mirror, the toilet bowl. Doubling up her right hand, she smashed the mirror to smithereens. Her husband removed the bathroom door and, gagging from the odor, placed her on the sofa bed on the porch, cleaned her off, then dressed her open wound, positioning a clean bag over the plastic rim that held it in place. "There," he said. "Everything's going to be all right. You're going to be just fine."

"I was brushing my hair," she said. "My hand slipped." He pulled mirror slivers out of her fist with tweezers, swabbed the cuts in her hand with witch hazel, saying, "There. That's better."

"Nothing you say or do will make me feel better," she said. She smelled the bile; tasted it at the back of her mouth. She ran her tongue along her teeth, convinced they had turned green. "I want my red bed jacket," she said. "Not this raggedy thing. Why didn't you bring me the red one?"

"I'm fixing tea," he said, running from the room. She heard him gag in the kitchen.

Anne Brashler, "He Read to Her," was originally published in *Iowa Woman*, reprinted in the anthology *Chicago Works*. Morton Press, Chicago, 1990. Reprinted by permission of the author's estate. Copyright © 1988 by Anne Brashler.

"I don't want tea!" she shouted. "Just leave me alone." The kettle whistled, playing an organ strain from Bach, sounding nervous. She knew he'd bring the tea, the double-crostics book, the reference books. She'd looked up the Down answers of the puzzle he'd been working on so that when he got stuck, she'd be able to provide the correct solution, shorten the game. He'd made a cherry wood bed tray, carved flowers around its edges, and was carrying it in, its legs splayed like a little dog flying. "Tea," he said. "Lemon slices, sugar; a rose for my beautiful wife."

"You creep," she said. "That's not going to do any good." She watched his face pale, contort, then smooth out like a person beatified. "I have something different today," he said. He held a book behind him like a surprise.

"Oh yeah?" she said. "It's a quote by Thomas Wolfe from *Look Home-ward, Angel*. The definition for Number One Down is 'geometric progres-sion.'" She wished she could hurt him but didn't know how; double-crostics was the best she could do.

"You looked," he said. "But that isn't it. I did that puzzle after you went to bed last night." He puffed pillows into shape, then tucked them under her head, ignoring her when she made her body stiffen. The bag gurgled as liquid hit the plastic.

"Why don't you just leave me alone?" she said and was instantly sorry. Lord knows it wasn't his fault. Lord knows. A joke. Lord, Lord, have mercy. Outside a squirrel chased a blue jay up a willow tree; blue and gray among silvery leaves. Their porch was over the garage, so in summer, with trees filled out, it felt as though they were in the branches of a forest. Their daughter had insisted she recuperate here, in this room, her favorite.

He sat down, ignoring her, then opened the book and began to read in a soft clear voice: "*Call me Ishmael. Some years ago—never mind how long precisely—having little or no money in my purse, and nothing particular to inter-est me on shore, I thought I would sail about a little and see the watery part of the world. . . .*" His face was intense, as if he'd turned into a priest since she'd been away.

"Are you going to read the whole damn book out loud?" she asked. She wondered if she'd be angry for the rest of her life. She'd hoped she'd be able to laugh again, say something nice once in a while.

"I thought I might," he said.

A breeze picked up leaves, turned them over, making different shades of green. The children had guests; they were racing with inner tubes in the pool. Her son had found huge truck tires at a flea market, hosed them off, patched the inner tubes with colored swatches. Her daughter had taken over the household chores while she'd been in the hospital. They'd kept the family running, shipshape. Her husband, too; he'd had a shock, nearly losing her, going out of his mind with guilt, with self-loathing, the worst kind of pain. "I'd like that, Darly," she finally said. The tea was cold but she drank it anyway.

"Say that again."

"Say what?"

"What you just said."

"Darly? I stole it from some story," she said. Her bag filled suddenly and she thought how convenient it all was.

"I like that. Call me that. Will you call me that?" he asked. He leaned forward, his gray head nestling in the hollow of her shoulder.

"But it's not mine," she said.

"I don't care. I like it."

"Some man said it to his wife. He called her that before they divorced." Was she threatening? Lord knows.

"I don't care," he said.

"Darly," she said, sighing. "Read to me." They'll sort it out later. When cheers for the winner of the inner tube race rose from the pool, she pretended the cheers were for her; she pretended she was a star.

". . . *Whenever I find myself growing grim about the mouth; whenever it is a damp, drizzly November in my soul . . .*" She lay back and closed her eyes. His voice was music; he became Ishmael, telling her a story.

PART III

Parents and Sick Children

Parents expect to take care of their children through the ordinary illnesses, accidents, and vagaries of childhood and adolescence. Sometimes, however, the demands of this sphere of caregiving go beyond what all parents experience into the realm of what no parent wants to endure. The three stories and two poems in this section illustrate such difficult caregiving situations.

In "How to Win," Rosellen Brown describes a mother whose young son, Christopher, is extremely hyperactive. "Watch Christopher take a room sometime; that's the word for it. Like an army subduing a deserted plain," she says. Her husband and their physician are not worried, but she is frightened by his uncontrollable outbursts. One day she follows him to kindergarten, where she learns a painful lesson about how others control his behavior.

Lorrie Moore's story "People Like That Are the Only People Here" is squarely in the medical arena. "'I've never heard of a baby having chemo,' the Mother says. Baby and Chemo, she thinks: they should never even appear in the same sentence together, let alone the same life." Baby has a kidney tumor and surgery to remove his kidney; Mother tries to adopt the look and attitude of the other Midwestern mothers of bald-headed little boys, "with their blond hair and sweatpants and sneakers and determined pleasantness." But she is different. "She knows, for instance, too many people in Greenwich Village." This story evokes strong feelings in many readers because of Moore's caustic portrayals of the people she meets in "Peed-Onk" (Pediatric Oncology). But every caregiver can resonate to this thought: "In the end you suffer alone. But at the beginning you suffer with a whole lot of others."

A more benign hospital atmosphere is evoked in Sarah Day's poem "Children's Ward." In this nighttime setting, "another world. / Like a pressurised aircraft at night / the hum insinuates itself into rows of dreams." Parents are "camped on cots like refugees." A mother strokes her baby's back, her "dulcet voice / sings out an aria—/ the two syllables of his name." Here mothers measure every breath with their soothing hands.

People suffering with a whole lot of others, in Moore's phrase, is the theme of "Parents Support Group," a poem by Dick Allen. The setting is a hospital where children who have attempted suicide or are anorexic are being treated. The therapist "Takes a long, long, long, long, *long* while / Before he starts, reluctantly. That hot potato, Pain, / Goes round and round the table." The group is made up of weeping strangers, brought together by their children, who "aimlessly . . . shot down our world."

Parents do not ordinarily expect to be caring for an adult child. The Iraq and Afghanistan wars have created a new army of family caregivers. "Starter" by Amy Hanridge is about a young Apache woman who served in the Marines and has come home to her mother and sister in Arizona. Unlike the other pieces in this section, the narrator is not Mama, the caregiver, but Kayla, the veteran. She was not physically wounded but has been emotionally damaged by her experiences. She understands what Mama expects and wants her to be like, but only with the help of a therapist can she even begin to deal with her isolation and confusion and link it to the Apache way of life.

23

How to Win

❧ *Rosellen Brown*

All they need at school is permission on a little green card that says, *Keep this child at bay. Muffle him, tie his hands, his arms to his ankles, anything at all. Distance, distance. Dose him.* And they gave themselves permission. They never even mentioned a doctor, and their own certified bureaucrat in tweed (does he keep a badge in his pocket like the cops?) drops by the school twice a year for half a day. But I insisted on a doctor. And did and did, had to, because Howard keeps repeating vaguely that he is "within the normal range of boyish activity."

"But I live with it, all day every day."

"It? Live with *it?*"

Well, Howard can be as holy as he likes, I am his mother and I will not say "him." Him is the part I know, Christopher my first child and first son, the boy who was a helpless warm mound once in a blue nightie tied at the bottom to keep his toes in. ("God, Margaret, you are dramatic and sentimental and sloppy. How about being realistic for a change?") "It" is what races around my room at night, a bat, pulling down the curtain cornice, knocking over the lamps, tearing the petals off the flowers and stomping them, real or fake, to a powder.

Watch Christopher take a room sometime; that's the word for it, like an army subduing a deserted plain. He stands in the doorway always for one extra split-split second, straining his shoulders down as though he's hitching himself to some machine, getting into harness. He has no hips, and round little six-year-old shoulders that look frail but are made of welded steel that has no give when you grab them. Then what does he see ahead of him? I'm no good at guessing. The room is an animal asleep, trusting the air, its last mistake. (See, I am sympathetic to the animal.) He leaps on it and leaves it disemboweled, then turns his dark eyes to me where I stand—when I stand, usually I'm dervishing around trying to stop the bloodshed—and they ask me, Where did it go? What happened? Who killed this thing, it was just breathing, I wanted to play with it. Christopher. When you're not here to look at me I have to laugh at your absurd powers. You are incontinent, you leak energy. As for me, I gave birth to someone else's child.

There is a brochure inside the brown bottle that the doctor assigned us, very gay, full-color, busy with children riding their bicycles right through patches of daffodils, sleeping square in the middle of their pillows, doing their homework with a hazy expression to be attributed to concentration, not medication. NONADDICTIVE! NO SIGNIFICANT SIDE EFFECTS! Dosage should decrease by or around puberty. Counterindications epilepsy, heart and circulatory complications, severe myopia and related eye problems. See *Journal of Pediatric Medicine*, III 136, F'71; *Pharmacology Bulletin*, v. 798, 18, pp. 19-26, D'72. CAUTION: DO NOT ALLOW CHILDREN ACCESS TO PILLS! SPECIAL FEATURE: U-LOK-IT CAP! REMEMBER, TEACH YOUR CHILD THE ETIQUETTE OF THE MEDICINE CABINET!

I know how he dreams me. I know because I dream his dreams. He runs to hide in me. Battered by the stick of the old dark, he comes fast, hic-coughing terror. By the time I am up, holding him, it has hobbled off, it must be, into his memory. I've pulled on a robe, I spread my arms—do they look winged or webbed?—to pull him out of himself, hide him, swear the witch is nowhere near. He doesn't go to his father. But he won't look at my face.

It was you! He looks up at me finally and says nothing, but I see him thinking. *So*: I was the witch, with a club behind my bent back. I the hundred-stalked flower with webbed branches. I with the flayed face held in my two hands like a bloody towel. Then how can I help him?

I whisper to him, wordless; just a music. He answers, "Mama." It is a faint knocking, through layers of dirt, through flowers.

His sister Jody will dream those dreams, and all the children who will follow her. I suppose she will, like chicken pox every child can expect them: there's a three o'clock in the dark night of children's souls too, let's not be too arrogant taking our prerogatives. But if she does, she'll dream them alone, no accomplices. I won't meet her halfway, give her my own last fillip, myself in shreds.

I've been keeping a sort of log: a day in the life. For no purpose, since my sense of futility runs deeper than any data can testify to. Still it cools me off.

He is playing with Jacqueline. They are in the Rosenbergs' yard. C. is on his way to the sandbox, which belongs to Jackie's baby brother, Brian, so I see trouble ahead. I will not interfere. No, intervene is the word they use. Interfere is not as objective, it's the mess that parents make, as opposed to the one the doctors make. As he goes down the long narrow yard at a good clip, C. pulls up two peonies, knocks over Brian's big blond blocky wooden horse (for which he has to stop and plant his feet very deliberately, it's that well-balanced, i.e., expensive). Kicks over short picket fence around tulips, finally gets to sandbox, walks up to Jackie, whose back is to him, and pushes her hard. She falls against fence and goes crying to her mother with a splinter. She doesn't even bother to retaliate, knowing him too well? Then he leans down into the sand. Turns to me again, that innocent face. It is not conniving or falsely naive, I swear it's not. He isn't that kind of clever. Nor is he a gruff bully boy who likes to fly from trees and conquer turf; he has a small peaked face, a little French, I think, in need of one of those common Gallic caps with the peak on the front; a narrow forehead on which his dark hair lies flat like a salon haircut. Anything but a bully, this helpless child of mine—he has a weird natural elegance that terrifies me, as though it is true, what I feel, that he was intended to be someone else. . . . Now he seems to be saying, Well, take all this stuff away if you don't want me to touch it. Get me out of this goddamn museum. Who says I'm not provoked? *That's what you say to each other.*

Why is *he* not glass? He will break us all without so much as chipping.

The worst thing I can think. I am dozing in the sun, Christopher is in kindergarten, Jody is napping, and I am guiltily trying to coax a little color into my late-fall pallor. It's a depressing bleary sun up there. But I sleep a little, waking in fits and snatches when Migdalia next door lets her kid have it and his whine sails across the yards, and when the bus shakes the earth all the way under the gas mains and water pipes to China. The worst thing is crawling through my head like a stream of red ants: What if he and I, Howie and I, had been somewhere else way back that night we smiled and nodded and made Christopher? If the night had been bone-cracking cold? If we were courting some aloneness, back to back? But it was summer, we'd been married three months, and the bottom sheet was spread like a picnic cloth. If there is an astrologer's clock, that's what we heard announcing to us the time was propitious; but I rehearse the time again. We lived off Riverside Drive that year and the next, I will float a thundercloud across the river from the Palisades and just as Howie turns to me I will have the most extraordinary burst of rain, sludgy and cold, explode through the open windows everywhere and finish us for the evening. The rugs are soaked, our books on the desk are corrugated with dampness, we snap at each other, Howie breaks a beer glass and blames me. We unmake him. . . . Another night we will make a different child. Don't the genes shift daily in their milky medium like lottery tickets in their fishbowl? I unmake Christopher's skin and bone: egg in the water, blind; a single sperm thrusts out of its soft side, retreating. Arrow swimming backwards, tail drags the heavy head away from life. All the probability in the universe cheers. He is unjoined. I wake in a clammy sweat. The sun, such as it was, is caught behind the smokestacks at the far end of Pacific Street. I feel dirty, as though I've sinned in my sleep, and there's that fine perpetual silt on my arms and legs and face, the Con Ed sunburn. I go in and start making lunch for Christopher, who will survive me.

❧

Log: He is sitting at the kitchen table trying to string kidney beans on a needle and thread. They do it in kindergarten. I forgot to ask why. Jody wakes upstairs, way at the back of the house with her door closed, and C. says quietly, without looking up from his string, "Ma, she's up." It's like hearing something happening, I don't know, a mile away. He has the instincts of an Indian guide, except when I stand right next to him to talk. Then it blows right by.

And when she's up. He seems to make a very special effort to be gentle with his little sister. I can see him forcibly subdue himself, tuck his hands inside his pockets or push them into the loops of his pants so that he loses no honor in restraint. But every now and then it gets the better of him. He walked by her just a minute ago and did just what he does to anything that's not nailed down or bigger than he is: gave her a casual but precise push. The way the bathmat slips into the tub without protest, the glass bowl gets smashed, its pieces settling with a resigned tinkle. I am, of course, the one who's resigned: I hear them ring against each other before they hit the ground, in the silence that envelops the shove.

This time Jody chose to lie back on the rug—fortunately it wasn't cement, I am grateful for small favors—and watch him. An amazing, endearing thing for a two-year-old. I think she has all the control that was meant for the two of them, and this is fair to neither. Eyes wide open, untearful, Jody, the antidote, was thinking something about her brother. She cannot say what.

When his dosage has been up a while, he begins to cringe before her. It is unpredictable and unimaginable but true, and I bear witness to it here.

As I was writing the above he ran in and hid behind my chair. Along came J., who had just righted herself after the attack on her; she was pulling her corn popper, vaguely humming. For C., an imagined assault? Provoked? Real? Wished for?

Howard, on his way out of the breakfast chaos, bears his briefcase like a shield, holds it in front of him for lack of space while he winds his way around the table in our little alcove, planting firm kisses on our foreheads. On his way out the door he can be expected to say something cheerful and blind to encourage me through the next unpredictable half hour before I walk Christopher up the block to school. This morning, unlocking the front gate, I caught him pondering. "Well, what are other kids like? I mean we've never had any others so how do we know where they fall on the spectrum?"

"We know," I said. "What about Jody?"

"Oh," he said, waving her away like a fly. "I mean boys."

"We also know because we're not knots on logs, some of us, that's how we know. What was it he did to your shaver this morning?"

Smashed it to smithereens is what he did, and left cobweb cracks in the mirror he threw it at.

To which his father shrugged and turned to pull the gate shut fast.

Why did we have Jody? People dare to ask, astonished, though it's none of their business. They mean, and expect us to forgive them, how could we take such a martyr's chance? I tell them that when C. was born I was ready for a large family. You can't be a secretary forever, no matter how many smash titles your boss edits. Nor an administrative assistant, nor an indispensable right hand. I've got my own arms, for which I need all the hands I've got. I like to be boss, thank you, in my own house. It's a routine by now, canned as an Alka-Seltzer ad.

But I'll tell you. For a long time I guarded very tensely against having another baby. C. was hurting me too much, already he was. Howard would rap with his fist on my nightgowned side, demanding admission. For a while I played virgin. I mean, I didn't try, I wasn't playing. He just couldn't make any headway. I've heard it called dys-something; also cross bones, to get right down to what it's like. (Dys-something puts me right in there with my son, doesn't it? I'll bet there's some drug, some muscle relaxant that bones you and just lays you out on the knife like a chicken to be stuffed and trussed. . . .) Even though it wasn't his fault I'll never forgive Howard for using his fists on me, even as gently and facetiously as he did. Finally I guess he got tired of trying to disarm me one night at a time, of bringing wine to bed or dancing with me obscenely like a kid at a petting party or otherwise trying to distract me while he stole up on me. So that's when he convinced me to have another baby. I guess it seemed easier. "We'll make Christopher our one exceptional child while we surround him with ordinary ones. We'll grow a goddamn garden around him, he'll be outnumbered."

Well—I bought it. We could make this child matter less. It was an old and extravagant solution. Black flowers in his brain, what blight would the next one have, I insisted he *promise* me. He lied, ah, he lied with his hand between my legs, he swore the next would be just as beautiful but timid— "Downright phlegmatic, how's that?"—and would teach Christopher to be human. So I sighed, desperate to believe, and unlocked my thighs, gone rusty and stiff. But I'll tell you, right as he turned out, by luck, to be, I think I never trusted him again, one of my two deceitful boys, because whatever abandon I once had is gone, sure as my waist is gone. I feel it now and Howard is punished for it. Starting right then, making Jody, I have dealt myself out in careful proportions, like an unreliable cook bent only on her batter.

Meanwhile I lose one lamp, half the ivory on the piano keys, and all my sewing patterns to my son in a single day. On the same day I lose my temper, lose it so irretrievably that I am tempted to pop one of Christopher's little red pills myself and go quietly. Who's the most frightening, the skimpy six-year-old flying around on the tail of his bird of prey, or his indispensable right-hand mama smashing the canned goods into the closet with a sound generally reserved for the shooting range? All the worse, off his habit for a few days, his eyes clear, his own, he is trying to be sweet, he smiles wanly whenever some catastrophe overtakes him, like an actor with no conviction. But someone else controls his muscles. He is not riding it now but lives in the beak of something huge and dark that dangles him just out of my reach.

Our brains are all circuitry; not very imaginative, I tend to see it blue and red and yellow like the wires in phones, easier to sort impulses that way. I want to see inside Christopher's head, I stare viciously though I try to do it when he's involved with something else. (He never is, he would feel me a hundred light years behind him.) I vow never to *study* him again, it's futile anyway, his forehead's not a one-way mirror. Promises, always my promises: they are glass. I know when they shatter—no, when he shatters them, throwing something of value—there will be edges to draw blood, edges everywhere. He says, "What are you *looking* at all the time? Bad Christopher the dragon?" He looks wilted, pathetic, seen-through. But I haven't seen a thing.

"Chrissie." I put my arms around him. He doesn't want to bruise the air he breathes, maybe we're all jumbled in his sight. He doesn't read yet, I know that's why. It's all upside down or somehow mixed together-cubist sight, is there such a thing? He sees my face and the top of my head, say, at the same time. Or everything looms at him, quivering like a fun-house mirror, swollen, then slowly disappears down to a point. He has to subdue it before it overtakes him? How would we ever know? Why, if he saw just what we see—the cool and calm of all the things of the world all sorted out like laundry ("Oh, Margaret, come off it!")—why would he look so bewildered most of the time, like a terrier being dragged around by his collar, his small face thrust forward into his own perpetual messes?

He comes to me just for a second, pulling on his tan wind-breaker, already breathing fast to run away somewhere, and while I hold him tight a minute, therapeutic hug for both of us, he pinches my arm until the purple capillaries dance with pain.

"Let me take him with me when I go to D.C. next week." Howard.

I stare at him. "You've got to be kidding."

"No, why would I kid about it? We'll manage, we can go see some buildings after my conference is out, go to the Smithsonian. He'd love the giant pendulum." His eyes are already there in the cool of the great vaulted room where everything echoes and everything can break. I am fascinated by his casualness. "What would he do all day while you're in your meeting? Friend. My intrepid friend."

"Oh, we'd manage something. He'd keep busy. Paper and pencil . . ."

"*Howie.*" Am I crazy? Is he? Do we live in the same house?

He comes and takes both my hands. There is that slightly conniving look my husband gets that makes me forget, goddammit, why I married him. He is all too reasonable and gentle a man most of the time, but this look is way in the back of his eyes behind a pillar, peeking out. I feel surrounded. "You can't take him." I wrench my hands away.

"Maggie—" and he tries to take them again, bungler, as though they're contested property.

"I forbid it. Insanity. You'll end up crushing him to death to get a little peace! I know."

He smiles with unbearable patience. "I know how to handle my son."

But I walk out of the room, thin-lipped, taking a bowl of fruit to the children who are raging around, both of them, in front of the grade-A educational television that's raging back.

The next week Howie goes to Washington and we all go to the airport to see him off. I don't know what Howard told him, but while Jody sleeps Christopher cries noisily in the back of the car and flings himself around so wildly, like a caged bear, that I have to stop the car on the highway shoulder and buckle him into his seat belt. "You will walk home," I threaten, calm because I can see the battle plan. He's got a little of his father in him; that should make me feel better.

He hisses at me and goes on crying, forcing the tears and walloping the back of my seat with his feet the whole way home.

Log: The long long walk to school. A block and a half. Most of the kids in kindergarten with Christopher walk past our house alone, solidly bearing straight west with the bland eight o'clock sun at their backs. They concentrate, they have been told not to cross heavy traffic alone, not to speak to strangers, not to dawdle. All the major wisdom of motherhood pinned to their jackets like a permission slip. Little orders turning into habits and hardening slowly to superego: an amber that holds commands forever. Christopher lacks it the way some children are born without a crucial body chemical. Therefore, I walk him to school every day, rain or shine, awake or asleep.

Jody's in her stroller, slouching. She'd rather be home. So would I. It's beginning to get chilly out, edgy, and that means the neighborhood's been stripped of summer and fall, as surely as if a man came by one day confiscating color. What little there is, you wouldn't think it could matter. Blame the mayor. The window boxes are crowded with brown stringy corpses, like tall crabgrass. Our noble pint-sized trees have shrunk back into themselves; they lose five years in winter. Fontaine, always improving his property, has painted his new brick wall silver over the weekend—it has a sepulchral gleam in the vague sunlight, twinkling as placidly as a woman who's come in sequins to a business meeting, *believing* in herself. Bless him. Next door to him the Rosenbergs have bought subtle aged wood shutters—they look like some dissected Vermont barn door—and a big rustic barrel that will stand achingly empty all winter, weighted with a hundred pounds of dirt to exhaust the barrel burglars. I wonder what my illusions look like through the front window.

Christopher's off and running. "Not in the street!" I get so tired of my voice, especially because I know he doesn't hear it. "Stay on the curb, Christopher." There's enough damage to be done there. He is swinging on that new couple's gate, straining the hinges, trying to fan up a good wind; then, when I look up from attending to Jody's dropped and splintered Ritz cracker, he's gone—clapping together two garbage can lids across the street. Always under an old lady's window, though with no particular joy—his job, it's there to be done. Jody is left with her stroller braked against a tree for safekeeping while I retrieve him. No one ever told me I'd grow up to be a shepherdess; and bad at it too—undone by a single sheep.

We are somehow at the corner, at least I can demand he hold my hand and drag us across the street where the crossing guard stands and winks at me daily, as dependably as a blinking light. She is a good lady, Mrs. Cortes, from a couple of blocks down in the projects, with many matching daughters, one son, Anibal, on the sixth-grade honor roll, and another on Riker's Island, a junkie. She is waving cars and people forward in waves, demonstrating "community involvement" to placate the gods who are seeing to Anibal's future, I know it. I recognize something deep behind her lively eyes, sunk there: a certain desperate casualness while the world has its way with her children. Another shepherdess without a chance. I give her my little salute.

By now, my feet heavy with the monotony of this trip, we are on the long school block. The barbed wire of the playground breaks for the entrance halfway down. This street, unlived on, is an unrelenting tangle—no one ever sees the generous souls who bequeath their dead cars to the children, but there are dozens, in various stages of decay; they must make regular deliveries. Christopher's castles; creative playthings, and broken already so he never gets blamed. For some reason he picks the third one. He's already in there, across a moat of broken windshield glass, reaching for the steering wheel. The back seat's burned out, the better to jump on. All the chrome has been cannibalized by the adults—everything that twists or lifts off, leaving a carcass of flung bones, its tin flesh dangling.

"Christopher, you are late and I. Am. Not. Waiting." But he will not come that way. My son demands the laying-on of hands. Before I can maneuver my way in, feeling middle-aged and worrying about my skirt, hiked up over my rear, he is tussling not with one boy but with two. They fight over nothing—just lock hands and wrestle as a kind of greeting. "I break the muh-fuh's head," one announces matter-of-factly—second grader maybe. Christopher doesn't fight for stakes like that, though. Whoever wants his head can have it, he's fighting to get his hands on something, keep them warm. I am reaching over the jagged door, which is split in two and full of rainwater. The school bell rings, that raspy grinding, and the two boys, with a whoop, leap over the downed windshield and are gone. Christopher is grater-scraped along one cheek, but we have arrived more or less in one piece.

I decide I'd better come in with him and see to it his cheek is washed off. He is, of course, long gone by the time I park the stroller and take the baby out. He never bothers to say good-bye. Maybe six-year-olds don't.

I pull open the heavy door to P.S. 193. It comes reluctantly, like it's in many parts. These doors are not for children. But then, neither is the school. . . . It's a fairly new building, but the 1939 World's Fair architecture has just about caught up with the lobby—those heavy streamlined effects.

A ship, that's what it looks like; a dated ocean liner, or the lobby of Rockefeller Center, one humble corner of it. What do the kids see, I wonder? Not grandeur.

There's a big lit-up case to the left that shows off sparse student pieties, untouchable as seven-layer cakes at the bakery. THIS LAND IS *Your* LAND, THIS LAND IS *My* LAND. Every figure in the pictures, brown, black, dead-white (blank), mustard yellow, tulip red and olive green (who's that?) is connected more or less at the wrist, like uncut paper dolls (HANDS ACROSS THE SEA). The whole world's afraid to drop hands, the hell with summit talks, SALT talks, we're on the buddy system. Well, they go up and down the halls irrevocably linked so, their lips sealed, the key thrown over their endless shoulder, only the teacher nattering on and on about discipline and respect, wearing heels that must sound like SS boots, though they are intended merely to mean business. Christopher tells me only that his teachers are noisy and hurt his ears; he does not bother to specify how.

And what he sees when he puts his thin shoulder to the door at 8:30 and heaves? He probably catches that glaring unnecessary shine on the floor, an invitation, and takes it. That worried crease between big eyes, his face looks back at him out of deep water. Deeper when he's drugged. So he careens around without ice skates, knocks against other kids hard, thumps into closed doors, nearly cracks open THIS LAND IS YOUR LAND. He is the wiseacre who dances to hold the door for his class, then when the last dark pigtail is through skips off in the wrong direction, leaps the steps to the gym or the auditorium or whatever lives down there in deserted silence most of the morning, the galley of this ship. I don't blame him, of course I don't, but that isn't the point, is it? I am deprived of these fashionable rebellious points. We only, madam, allow those in control to be out of control. As it were. If you follow. Your son, madam, is not rebelling. He is unable. Is beyond. Is utterly. Is unthinkable. Catch him before we do.

We are certainly late, the lines are all gone, the kids settling into their rooms, their noise dwindling like a cut-back motor. Jody and I just stand for a minute or two tuning in. Her head is heavy on my shoulder. Already there's a steady monitor traffic, the officious kids scurrying to do their teachers' bidding like tailless mice. I was one of them for years and years, God, faceless and obliging: official blackboard eraser (which meant a few cool solitary minutes just before three each day, down in the basement storeroom clapping two erasers together, hard, till they smoked with the day's vanished lessons). I would hardly have stopped my frantic do-gooding to give the time of day (off the clocks that jerked forward with a click every new minute) to the likes of Christopher. I'd have given him a wide berth, I can see myself going the other way if I saw him coming toward me in the narrow hall.

This hall, just like the ones I grew up in except for the "modernistic" shower tile that reaches halfway up, has a muted darkened feeling, an underwater thrum. Even the tile is like the Queens Midtown Tunnel, deserted. I will not be particularly welcome in Christopher's kindergarten room; there is that beleaguered proprietary feeling that any parent is a spy or come to complain. (I, in my own category, have been forbidden to complain, at least tacitly, having been told that my son really needs one whole teacher to himself, if not for his sake, then for the safety of the equipment and "the consumables," of which he is not one.)

Christopher has disappeared into his class which—I see it through the little porthole—is neat and earnest and not so terribly different from a third-grade room, say, with its alphabets and exhortations to patriotism and virtue above eye level. They are allowed to paint in one color at a time. A few, I see, have graduated to two; they must be disciplined, promising children in their securely tied smocks. One spring they will hatch into monitors. Christopher is undoubtedly banned from the painting corner. (Classroom economy? Margaret, your kitchen, your bedroom, your bathroom this morning. Searching for the glass mines hidden between the tiles.) Mrs. Seabury is inspecting hands. The children turn them, patty-cake, and step back when she finishes her scrutiny, which is as grave as a doctor's. Oh Christopher! She has sent him and another little boy to the sink to scrub; to throw water, that is, and stick their fingers in the spout in order to shower the children in the back of the room. I am not going in there to identify myself.

Mrs. Seabury is the kind of teacher who, with all her brown and black kids on one side of the room (this morning in the back, getting showered), talks about discrimination and means big from little, forward from backward, ass from elbow. Now I see she has made Christopher an honorary Black child, or maybe one of your more rambunctious Puerto Ricans. They are all massed back there for the special inattention of the aide, who is one of my least favorite people: she is very young and wears a maxi skirt that the kids keep stepping on when she bends down. (Therefore she bends down as little as possible.) The Future Felons of America and their den mother. I'm caught somewhere between my first flash of anger and then shame at what I suppose, wearily, is arrogance. What am I angry at? That he has attained pariah-hood with them, overcoming his impeccable WASP heritage in a single leap of adrenaline? Jesus. They are the "unruly characters" he's supposed to be afraid of: latchkey babies, battered boys and abused girls, or loved but hungry, scouted by rats while they sleep. Products of this-and-that converging, social, political, economic, each little head impaled on a point of the grid. Christopher? My warm, healthy, nursed and coddled, vitamin-enriched boy, born on Blue Cross, swaddled in his grandparents' gifts from Lord & Taylor? What in the hell is our excuse? My pill-popping baby, so sad, so reduced and taken from himself when he's on, so indescribable, airborne, when he's off. This week he is off; I am sneaking him a favor.

I see him now flapping around in a sort of ragged circle with the other unimaginables, under the passive eye of that aide. Crows? Buzzards? Not pigeons, anyway. They make their own rowdy music. Then Christopher clenches his whole body—I see it coming—and stops short, slamming half a dozen kids together, solid rear-end collisions. It looks like the New Jersey Turnpike, everybody whiplashed, tumbling down. No reason, no whys, there is never anything to explain. Was the room taking off, spinning him dizzy? Was he fending something off, or trying to catch hold? The others turn to him, shout so loud I can hear them out here where I'm locked, underwater—and they all pile on. Oh, can they pile! It's a sport in itself. Feet and hands and dark faces deepening a shade. The aide gets out of the way, picking her skirt out of the rubble of children at her feet.

One heavy dark boy with no wrists finally breaks through the victor: his foot is on Christopher's neck. The little pale face jerks up stiffly, like an executed man's. I turn away. When I make myself turn back the crowd is unraveling as Mrs. Seabury approaches. Faces all around are taking on that half-stricken, half-delighted "uh-oh" look. I was always good at that, one of the leaders of censure and shock. It felt good.

But Christopher sinks down, quiet. She reaches down roughly and yanks his fresh white collar. Good boy, he doesn't look up at her. But something is broken. The mainspring, the defiant arch of his back that I would recognize, his, mine, I find I am weeping, soundless as everything around me, I feel it suddenly like blood on my cheeks. This teacher, this stranger and her cohorts have him by his pale limp neck. They are teaching him how to lose; or me how to win. My son is down for the count, breathing comfortably, accommodating, only his fingers twitching fiercely at his sides like gill slits puffing, while I stand outside, a baby asleep on my shoulder. I am the traitor, he sees me through my one-way mirror, and he is right. I am the witch. Every day they walk on his neck, I see that now, but he will never tell me about it. I weep but cannot move.

24

People Like That
Are the Only People Here

❧ *Lorrie Moore*

A beginning, an end: there seems to be neither. The whole thing is like a cloud that just lands, and everywhere inside it is full of rain. A start: the Mother finds a blood clot in the Baby's diaper. What is the story? Who put this here? It is big and bright, with a broken, khaki-colored vein in it. Over the weekend, the Baby had looked listless and spacey, clayey and grim. But today he looks fine—so what is this thing, startling against the white diaper, like a tiny mouse heart packed in snow? Perhaps it belongs to someone else. Perhaps it is something menstrual, something belonging to the Mother or to the Babysitter, something the Baby has found in a wastebasket and for his own demented baby reasons stowed away here. (Babies— they're crazy! What can you do?) In her mind, the Mother takes this away from his body and attaches it to someone else's. There. Doesn't that make more sense?

Still, she phones the children's hospital clinic. Blood in the diaper, she says, and, sounding alarmed and perplexed, the woman on the other end says, "Come in now."

Such pleasingly instant service! Just say "blood." Just say "diaper." Look what you get!

In the examination room, the pediatrician, the nurse, and the head resident all seem less alarmed and perplexed than simply perplexed. At first, stupidly, the Mother is calmed by this. But soon, besides peering and saying "Hmm," the doctor, the nurse, and the head resident are all drawing their mouths in, bluish and tight—morning glories sensing noon. They fold their arms across their white-coated chests, unfold them again, and jot things down. They order an ultrasound. Bladder and kidneys. Here's the card. Go downstairs, turn left.

In Radiology, the Baby stands anxiously on the table, naked against the Mother, as she holds him still against her legs and waist, the Radiologist's cold scanning disk moving about the Baby's back. The Baby whimpers, looks up at the Mother. *Let's get out of here*, his eyes beg. *Pick me up!* The Radiologist stops, freezes one of the many swirls of oceanic gray, and clicks repeatedly, a single moment within the long, cavernous weather map that is the Baby's insides.

"Are you finding something?" asks the Mother. Last year, her Uncle Larry had a kidney removed for something that turned out to be benign. These imaging machines! They are like dogs, or metal detectors: they find everything but don't know what they've found. That's where the surgeons come in. They're like the owners of the dogs. *Give me that*, they say to the dog. *What the heck is that?*

"The surgeon will speak to you," says the Radiologist.

"Are you finding something?"

"The surgeon will speak to you," the Radiologist says again. "There seems to be something there, but the surgeon will talk to you about it."

"My uncle once had something on his kidney," says the Mother. "So they removed the kidney and it turned out the something was benign."

The Radiologist smiles a broad, ominous smile. "That's always the way it is," he says. "You don't know exactly what it is until it's in the bucket."

"In the bucket," the Mother repeats.

"That's doctor talk," the Radiologist says.

"It's very appealing," says the Mother. "It's a very appealing way to talk." Swirls of bile and blood, mustard and maroon in a pail, the colors of an African flag or some exuberant salad bar: *in the bucket*—she imagines it all.

"The surgeon will see you soon," he says again. He tousles the Baby's ringlety hair. "Cute kid," he says.

Let's see now," says the Surgeon, in one of his examining rooms. He has stepped in, then stepped out, then come back in again. He has crisp, frowning features, sharp bones, and a tennis-in-Bermuda tan. He crosses his blue-cottoned legs. He is wearing clogs.

The Mother knows her own face is a big white dumpling of worry. She is still wearing her long, dark parka, holding the Baby, who has pulled the hood up over her head because he always thinks it's funny to do that. Though on certain windy mornings she would like to think she could look vaguely romantic like this, like some French Lieutenant's Woman of the Prairie, in all her saner moments she knows she doesn't. She knows she looks ridiculous—like one of those animals made out of twisted party balloons. She lowers the hood and slips one arm out of the sleeve. The Baby wants to get up and play with the light switch. He fidgets, fusses, and points.

"He's big on lights these days," explains the Mother.

"That's O.K," says the Surgeon, nodding toward the light switch. "Let him play with it." The Mother goes and stands by it, and the Baby begins turning the lights off and on, off and on.

"What we have here is a Wilms' tumor," says the Surgeon, suddenly plunged into darkness. He says "tumor" as if it were the most normal thing in the world.

"Wilms'?" repeats the Mother. The room is quickly on fire again with light, then wiped dark again. Among the three of them here there is a long silence, as if it were suddenly the middle of the night. "Is that apostrophe 's' or 's' apostrophe?" the Mother says finally. She is a writer and a teacher. Spelling can be important—perhaps even at a time like this, though she has never before been at a time like this, so there are barbarisms she could easily commit without knowing.

The lights come on; the world is doused and exposed.

" 'S' apostrophe," says the Surgeon. "I think." The lights go back out, but the Surgeon continues speaking in the dark. "A malignant tumor of the left kidney."

Wait a minute. Hold on here. The Baby is only a baby, fed on organic applesauce and soy milk—a little prince!—and he was standing so close to her during the ultrasound. How could he have this terrible thing? It must have been *her* kidney. A fifties kidney. A DDT kidney. The Mother clears her throat. "Is it possible it was my kidney on the scan? I mean, I've never heard of a baby with a tumor, and, frankly, I was standing very close." She would make the blood hers, the tumor hers; it would all be some treacherous, farcical mistake.

"No, that's not possible," says the Surgeon. The light goes back on.

"It's not?" says the Mother. Wait until it's *in the bucket*, she thinks. Don't be so sure. *Do we have to wait until it's in the bucket to find out a mistake has been made?*

"We will start with a radical nephrectomy," says the Surgeon, instantly thrown into darkness again. His voice comes from nowhere and everywhere at once. "And then we'll begin with chemotherapy after that. These tumors usually respond very well to chemo."

"I've never heard of a baby having chemo," the Mother says. Baby and Chemo, she thinks: they should never even appear in the same sentence together, let alone the same life. In her other life, her life before this day, she was a believer in alternative medicine. Chemotherapy? Unthinkable. Now, suddenly, alternative medicine seems the wacko maiden aunt to the Nice Big Daddy of Conventional Treatment. How quickly the old girl faints and gives way, leaves one just standing there. Chemo? Of course: chemo! Why, by all means: chemo. Absolutely! Chemo!

The Baby flicks the switch back on, and the walls reappear, big wedges of light checkered with small framed watercolors of the local lake. The Mother has begun to cry: all of life has led her here, to this moment. After this there is no more life. There is something else, something stumbling and unlivable, something mechanical, something for robots, but not life. Life has been taken and broken, quickly, like a stick. The room goes dark again, so that the Mother can cry more freely. How can a baby's body be stolen so fast? How much can one heaven-sent and unsuspecting child endure? Why has he not been spared this inconceivable fate?

Perhaps, she thinks, she is being punished: too many babysitters too early on. ("Come to Mommy! Come to MommyBabysitter!" she used to say. But it was a joke!) Her life, perhaps, bore too openly the marks and wigs of deepest drag. Her unmotherly thoughts had all been noted: the panicky hope that his nap would last just a little longer than it did; her occasional desire to kiss him passionately on the mouth (to make out with her baby!); her ongoing complaints about the very vocabulary of motherhood, how it degraded the speaker. ("Is this a poopie onesie? Yes, it's a very poopie onesie!") She had, moreover, on three occasions used the formula bottles as flower vases. She twice let the Baby's ears get fudgy with wax. A few afternoons last month, at snack time, she placed a bowl of Cheetos on the floor for him to eat, like a dog. She let him play with the Dustbuster. Just once, before he was born, she said, "Healthy? I just want the kid to be rich." A joke, for God's sake. After he was born, she announced that her life had become a daily sequence of mind-wrecking chores, the same ones over and over again, like a novel by Mrs. Camus. Another joke! These jokes will kill you. She had told too often, and with too much enjoyment, the story of how the Baby had said "Hi" to his high chair, waved at the lake waves, shouted "Goody-goody-goody" in what seemed to be a Russian accent, pointed at his eyes and said "Ice." And all that nonsensical baby talk: wasn't it a stitch? *Canonical babbling*, the language experts called it. He recounted whole stories in it, totally made up, she could tell; he embroidered, he fished, he exaggerated. What a card! To friends she spoke of his eating habits (carrots yes, tuna no). She mentioned, too much, his sidesplitting giggle. Did she have to be so boring? Did she have no consideration for others, for the intellectual demands and courtesies of human society? Would she not even attempt to be more interesting? It was a crime against the human mind not even to try.

Now her baby, for all these reasons—lack of motherly gratitude, motherly judgment, motherly proportion—will be taken away.

The room is fluorescently ablaze again. The Mother digs around in her parka pocket and comes up with a Kleenex. It is old and thin, like a mashed flower saved from a dance; she dabs it at her eyes and nose.

"The baby won't suffer as much as you," says the Surgeon.

And who can contradict? Not the Baby, who in his Slavic Betty Boop voice can say only *mama, dada, cheese, ice, byebye, outside, boogie-boogie, goody-goody, eddy-eddy,* and *car.* (Who is Eddy? They have no idea.) This will not suffice to express his mortal suffering. Who can say what babies do with their agony and shock? Not they themselves. (Baby talk: isn't it a stitch?) They put it all no place anyone can really see. They are like a different race, a different species: they seem not to experience pain the way we do. Yeah, that's it: their nervous systems are not as fully formed, and *they just don't experience pain the way we do.* A tune to keep one humming through the war. "You'll get through it," the Surgeon says.

"How?" asks the Mother. "How does one get through it?"

"You just put your head down and go," says the Surgeon. He picks up his file folder. He is a skilled manual laborer. The tricky emotional stuff is not to his liking. The babies. The babies! What can be said to console the parents about the babies? "I'll go phone the oncologist on duty to let him know," he says, and leaves the room.

"Come here, sweetie," the Mother says to the Baby, who has toddled off toward a gum wrapper on the floor. "We've got to put your jacket on." She picks him up and he reaches for the light switch again. Light, dark. Peekaboo: Where's baby? Where did baby go?

At home, she leaves a message—Urgent! Call me!—for the Husband on his voice mail. Then she takes the Baby upstairs for his nap, rocks him in the rocker. The Baby waves goodbye to his little bears, then looks toward the window and says, "Bye-bye, outside." He has, lately, the habit of waving goodbye to everything, and now it seems as if he sensed some imminent departure, and it breaks her heart to hear him. *Bye-bye!* She sings low and monotonously, like a small appliance, which is how he likes it. He is drowsy, dozy, drifting off. He has grown so much in the last year he hardly fits in her lap anymore; his limbs dangle off like a Pietà. His head rolls slightly inside the crook of her arm. She can feel him falling backward into sleep, his mouth round and open like the sweetest of poppies. All the lullabies in the world, all the melodies threaded through with maternal melancholy now become for her—abandoned as mothers can be by working men and napping babies—the songs of hard, hard grief. Sitting there, bowed and bobbing, the Mother feels the entirety of her love as worry and heartbreak. A quick and irrevocable alchemy: there is no longer one unworried scrap left for happiness. "If you go," she keens low into his soapy neck, into the ranunculus coil of his ear, "we are going with you. We are nothing without you. Without you, we are a heap of rocks. Without you, we are two stumps, with nothing any longer in our hearts. Wherever this takes you, we are following; we will be there. Don't be scared. We are going, too, wherever you go. That is that. That is that."

"Take notes," says the Husband, after coming straight home from work, midafternoon, hearing the news, and saying all the words out loud—*surgery, metastasis, dialysis, transplant*—then collapsing in a chair in tears. "Take notes. We are going to need the money."

"Good God," cries the Mother. Everything inside her suddenly begins to cower and shrink, a thinning of bones. Perhaps this is a soldier's readiness, but it has the whiff of death and defeat. It feels like a heart attack, a failure of will and courage, a power failure: a failure of everything. Her face, when she glimpses it in a mirror, is cold and bloated with shock, her eyes scarlet and shrunk. She has already started to wear sunglasses indoors, like a celebrity widow. From where will her own strength come? From some philosophy? From some frigid little philosophy? She is neither stalwart nor realistic and has trouble with basic concepts, such as the one that says events move in one direction only and do not jump up, turn around, and take themselves back.

The Husband begins too many of his sentences with "What if." He is trying to piece everything together, like a train wreck. He is trying to get the train to town.

"We'll just take all the steps, move through all the stages. We'll go where we have to go, we'll hunt, we'll find, we'll pay what we have to pay. What if we can't pay?"

"Sounds like shopping."

"I cannot believe this is happening to our little boy," he says, and starts to sob again.

What is to be said? You turn just slightly and there it is: the death of your child. It is part symbol, part devil, and in your blind spot all along, until it is upon you. Then it is a fierce little country abducting you; it holds you squarely inside itself like a cellar room, the best boundaries of you are the boundaries of it. Are there windows? Sometimes aren't there windows?

The Mother is not a shopper. She hates to shop, is generally bad at it, though she does like a good sale. She cannot stroll meaningfully through anger, denial, grief, and acceptance. She goes straight to bargaining and stays there. How much? She calls out to the ceiling, to some makeshift construction of holiness she has desperately though not uncreatively assembled in her mind and prayed to; a doubter, never before given to prayer, she must now reap what she has not sown; she must reassemble an entire altar of worship and begging. She tries for noble abstractions, nothing too anthropomorphic, just some Higher Morality, though if this particular Highness looks something like the Manager at Marshall Field's, sucking a Frango mint, so be it. Amen. Just tell me what you want, requests the Mother. And how do you want it? More charitable acts? A billion, starting now. Charitable thoughts? Harder, but of course! Of course! I'll do the cooking, honey, I'll pay the rent. Just tell me. *Excuse me?* Well, if not to you, to whom do I speak? Hello? To whom do I have to speak around here? A higher-up? A superior? Wait? I can wait. I've got the whole damn day.

The Husband now lies next to her on their bed, sighing. "Poor little guy could survive all this only to be killed in a car crash at the age of sixteen," he says.

The Mother, bargaining, considers this. "We'll take the car crash," she says.

"What?"

"Let's Make a Deal! Sixteen is a full life! We'll take the car crash. We'll take the car crash in front of which Carol Merrill is now standing."

Now the Manager of Marshall Field's reappears. "To take the surprises out is to take the life out of life," he says.

The phone rings. The Husband leaves the room.

"But I don't want these surprises," says the Mother." Here! You take these surprises!"

"To know the narrative in advance is to turn yourself into a machine," the Manager continues. "What makes humans human is precisely that they do not know the future. That is why they do the fateful and amusing things they do: who can say how anything will turn out? Therein lies the only hope for redemption, discovery, and—let's be frank—fun, fun, fun! There might be things people will get away with. And not just motel towels. There might be great illicit loves, enduring joy—or faith-shaking accidents with farm machinery. But you have to not know in order to see what stories your life's efforts bring you. The mystery is all."

The Mother, though shy, has grown confrontational. "Is this the kind of bogus, random crap they teach at merchandising school? We would like fewer surprises, fewer efforts and mysteries, thank you. K through 8; can we just get K through 8?" It now seems like the luckiest, most beautiful, most musical phrase she's ever heard: K through 8—the very lilt. The very thought.

The Manager continues, trying things out. "I mean, the whole conception of 'the story,' of cause and effect, the whole idea that people have a clue as to how the world works, is just a piece of laughable metaphysical colonialism perpetrated upon the wild country of time."

Did they own a gun? The Mother begins looking through drawers.

The Husband comes back in the room and observes her. "Ha! The Great Havoc That Is the Puzzle of All Life!" he says of the Marshall Field's management policy. He has just gotten off a conference call with the insurance company and the hospital. The surgery will be Friday. "It's all just some dirty capitalist's idea of a philosophy."

"Maybe it's just a fact of narrative, and you really can't politicize it," says the Mother. It is now only the two of them.

"Whose side are you on?"

"I'm on the Baby's side."

"Are you taking notes for this?"

"No."

"You're not?"

"No. I can't. Not this! I write fiction. This isn't fiction."

"Then write nonfiction. Do a piece of journalism. Get two dollars a word."

"Then it has to be true and full of information. I'm not trained. I'm not that skilled. Plus, I have a convenient personal principle about artists' not abandoning art. One should never turn one's back on a vivid imagination. Even the whole memoir thing annoys me."

"Well, make things up but pretend they're real."

"I'm not that insured."

"You're making me nervous."

"Sweetie, darling, I'm not that good. I can't *do this*. I can do—what can I do? I can do quasi-amusing phone dialogue. I can do succinct descriptions of weather. I can do screwball outings with the family pet. Sometimes I can do those. Honey, I only do what I can. I do *the careful ironies of daydream*. I do *the marshy ideas upon which intimate life is built*. But this? Our baby with cancer? I'm sorry. My stop was two stations back. This is irony at its most gaudy and careless. This is a Hieronymus Bosch of facts and figures and blood and graphs. This is a nightmare of narrative slop. This cannot be designed. This cannot even be noted in preparation for a design—"

"We're going to need the money."

"To say nothing of the moral boundaries of pecuniary recompense in a situation such as this—"

"What if the other kidney goes? What if he needs a transplant? Where are the moral boundaries there? What are we going to do, have bake sales?"

"We can sell the house. I hate this house. It makes me crazy."

"And we'll live—where, again?"

"The Ronald McDonald place. I hear it's nice. It's the least McDonald's can do."

"You have a keen sense of justice."

"I try. What can I say?"

The Husband buries his face in his hands: "Our poor baby. How did this happen to him?" He looks over and stares at the bookcase that serves as their nightstand. "And is any one of these baby books a help?" He picks up the Leach, the Spock, the "What to Expect." "Where in the pages or index of any of these does it say 'chemotherapy' or 'Hickman catheter' or 'renal sarcoma'? Where does it say 'carcinogenesis' or 'metastasis'? You know what these books are obsessed with? *Holding a fucking spoon.*" He begins hurling the books off the nightstand and against the far wall.

"Hey," says the Mother, trying to soothe. "Hey, hey, hey." But, compared with his stormy roar, her words are those of a backup singer—a Shondell, a Pip—a doo-wop ditty. Books, and now more books, continue to fly.

TAKE NOTES.

Is "fainthearted" one word or two? Student prose has wrecked her spelling.

It's one word. Two words—faint hearted—what would that be? The name of a drag queen.

TAKE NOTES.

In the end you suffer alone. But at the beginning you suffer with a whole lot of others. When your child has cancer you are instantly whisked away to another planet: one of bald-headed little boys. Pediatric Oncology. Peed-Onk. You wash your hands for thirty seconds in antibacterial soap before you are allowed to enter through the swinging doors. You put paper slippers on your shoes. You keep your voice down. "Almost all the children are boys," one of the nurses says." No one knows why. It's been documented, but a lot of people out there still don't realize it." The little boys are all from sweet-sounding places, Janesville and Appleton—little heartland towns with giant landfills, agricultural runoff, paper factories, Joe McCarthy's grave. (Alone a site of great toxicity, thinks the Mother. The soil should be tested.)

All the bald little boys look like brothers. They wheel their I.V.s up and down the single corridor of Peed-Onk. Some of the lively ones, feeling good for a day, ride the lower bars of their I.V.s while their large, cheerful mothers whizz them along the halls. *Wheee!*

The Mother does not feel large and cheerful. In her mind she is scathing, acid-tongued, wraith-thin, and chain-smoking out on a fire escape somewhere. Below her lie the gentle undulations of the Midwest, with all its aspirations to be—to be what? To be Long Island. How it has succeeded! Strip mall upon strip mall. Lurid water, poisoned potatoes. The Mother drags deeply, blowing clouds of smoke out over the disfigured cornfields. When a baby gets cancer, it seems stupid ever to have given up smoking. When a baby gets cancer, you think, Whom are we kidding? Let's all light up. When a baby gets cancer, you think, Who came up with *this* idea? What celestial abandon gave rise to *this?* Pour me a drink, so I can refuse to toast.

The Mother does not know how to be one of these other mothers, with their blond hair and sweatpants and sneakers and determined pleasantness. She does not think that she can be anything similar. She does not feel remotely like them. She knows, for instance, too many people in Greenwich Village. She mail-orders oysters and tiramisu from a shop in SoHo. She is close friends with four actual homosexuals. Her husband is asking her to Take Notes.

Where do these women get their sweatpants? She will find out.

She will start, perhaps, with the costume and work from there.

She will live according to the bromides: Take one day at a time. Take a positive attitude. *Take a hike!* She wishes that there were more interesting things that were useful and true, but it seems now that it's only the boring things that are useful and true. *One day at a time.* And *At least we have our health.* How ordinary. How obvious. One day at a time: you need a brain for that?

While the Surgeon is fine-boned, regal, and laconic—they have correctly guessed his game to be doubles—there is a bit of the mad, overcaffeinated scientist to the Oncologist. He speaks quickly. He knows a lot of studies and numbers. He can do the math. Good! Someone should be able to do the math! "It's a fast but wimpy tumor," he explains. "It typically metastasizes to the lung." He rattles off some numbers, time frames, risk statistics. Fast but wimpy: the Mother tries to imagine this combination of traits, tries to think and think, and can only come up with Claudia Osk from the fourth grade, who blushed and almost wept when called on in class but in gym could outrun everyone in the quarter-mile, fire-door-to-fence dash. The Mother thinks now of this tumor as Claudia Osk. They are going to get Claudia Osk, make her sorry. All right! Claudia Osk must die. Though it has never been mentioned before, it now seems clear that Claudia Osk should have died long ago. Who was she, anyway? So conceited, not letting anyone beat her in a race. Well, hey, hey, hey—don't look now, Claudia!

The Husband nudges her. "Are you listening?"

"The chances of this happening even just to one kidney are one in fifteen thousand. Now, given all these other factors, the chances on the second kidney are about one in eight."

"One in eight," says the Husband. "Not bad. As long as it's not one in fifteen thousand."

The Mother studies the trees and fish along the ceiling's edge in the Save the Planet wallpaper border. Save the Planet. Yes! But the windows in this very building don't open, and diesel fumes are leaking into the ventilating system, near which, outside, a delivery truck is parked. The air is nauseous and stale.

"Really," the Oncologist is saying, "of all the cancers he could get, this is probably one of the best."

"We win," says the Mother.

"'Best,' I know, hardly seems the right word. Look, you two probably need to get some rest. We'll see how the surgery and histology go. Then we'll start with chemo the week following. A little light chemo: vincristine and—"

"Vincristine?" interrupts the Mother. "Wine of Christ?"

"The names are strange, I know. The other one we use is actinomycin-D. Sometimes called dactinomycin. People move the 'D' around to the front."

"They move the 'D' around to the front," repeats the Mother.

"Yup," the Oncologist says. "I don't know why, they just do!"

"Christ didn't survive his wine," says the Husband.

"But of course he did," says the Oncologist and nods toward the Baby, who has now found a cupboard full of hospital linens and bandages and is yanking them all out onto the floor. "I'll see you guys tomorrow, after the surgery." And with that the Oncologist leaves.

"Or, rather, Christ was his wine," mumbles the Husband. Everything he knows about the New Testament he has gleaned from the soundtrack of *Godspell*. "His blood was the wine. What a great beverage idea."

"A little light chemo. Don't you like that one?" says the Mother. "*Eine kleine* dactinomycin. I'd like to see Mozart write that one up for a big wad o' cash."

"Come here, honey," the Husband says to the Baby, who has now pulled off both his shoes.

"It's bad enough when they refer to medical science as an inexact science," says the Mother. "But when they start referring to it as an art I get extremely nervous."

"Yeah. If we wanted art, Doc, we'd go to an art museum." The Husband picks up the Baby. "You're an artist," he says to the Mother with the taint of accusation in his voice. "They probably think you find creativity reassuring."

The Mother sighs. "I just find it inevitable. Let's go get something to eat." And so they take the elevator to the cafeteria, where there is a high chair, and where, not noticing, they all eat a lot of apples with the price tags still on them.

Because his surgery is not until tomorrow, the Baby likes the hospital. He likes the long corridors, down which he can run. He likes everything on wheels. The flower carts in the lobby! ("Please keep your boy away from the flowers," says the vender. "We'll buy the whole display," snaps the Mother, adding, "Actual children in a children's hospital—unbelievable, isn't it?") The Baby likes the other little boys. Places to go! People to see! Rooms to wander into! There is Intensive Care. There is the Trauma Unit. The Baby smiles and waves. What a little Cancer Personality! Bandaged citizens smile and wave back. In Peed-Onk there are the bald little boys to play with. Joey, Eric, Tim, Mort, and Tod. (Mort! Tod!) There is the four-year-old, Ned, holding his little deflated rubber ball, the one with the intriguing curling hose. The Baby wants to play with it. "It's mine, leave it alone," says Ned. "Tell the baby to leave it alone."

"Baby, you've got to share," says the Mother from a chair some feet away.

Suddenly, from down near the Tiny Tim Lounge, comes Ned's mother, large and blond and sweatpanted. "Stop that! Stop it!" she cries out, dashing toward the Baby and Ned and pushing the Baby away. "Don't touch that!" she barks at the Baby, who is only a baby and bursts into tears because he has never been yelled at like this before.

Ned's mom glares at everyone. "This is drawing fluid from Neddy's liver!" She pats at the rubber thing and starts to cry a little.

"Oh, my God," says the Mother. She comforts the Baby, who is also crying. She and Ned, the only dry-eyed people, look at each other. "I'm so sorry," she says to Ned and then to his mother. "I'm so stupid. I thought they were squabbling over a toy."

"It does look like a toy," agrees Ned. He smiles. He is an angel. All the little boys are angels. Total, sweet, bald little angels, and now God is trying to get them back for himself. Who are they, mere mortal women, in the face of this, this powerful and overwhelming and inscrutable thing, God's will? They are the mothers, that's who. You can't have him! they shout every day. You dirty old man! *Get out of here! Hands off!*

"I'm so sorry," says the Mother again. "I didn't know."

Ned's mother smiles vaguely. "Of course you didn't know," she says, and walks back to the Tiny Tim Lounge.

The Tiny Tim Lounge is a little sitting area at the end of the PeedOnk corridor. There are two small sofas, a table, a rocking chair, a television, and a VCR. There are various videos: "Speed," "Dune," "Star Wars." On one of the lounge walls there is a gold plaque with the musician Tiny Tim's name on it: years ago, his son was treated at this hospital, and so he donated money for this lounge. It is a cramped little lounge, which one suspects would be larger if Tiny Tim's son had actually lived. Instead, he died here, at this hospital, and now there is this tiny room which is part gratitude, part generosity, part *Fuck you*.

Sifting through the videocassettes, the Mother wonders what science fiction could begin to compete with the science fiction of cancer itself: a tumor, with its differentiated muscle and bone cells, a clump of wild nothing and its mad, ambitious desire to be something—something inside you, instead of you, another organism but with a monster's architecture, a demon's sabotage and chaos. Think of leukemia, a tumor diabolically taking liquid form, the better to swim about incognito in the blood. George Lucas, direct that!

Sitting with the other parents in the Tiny Tim Lounge, the night before the surgery, having put the Baby to bed in his high steel crib two rooms down, the Mother begins to hear the stories: leukemia in kindergarten, sarcomas in Little League, neuroblastomas discovered at summer camp. *Eric slid into third base, but then the scrape didn't heal.* The parents pat one another's forearms and speak of other children's hospitals as if they were resorts. "You were at St. Jude's last winter? So were we. What did you think of it? We loved the staff." Jobs have been quit, marriages hacked up, bank accounts ravaged; the parents have seemingly endured the unendurable. They speak not of the *possibility* of comas brought on by the chemo but of the *number* of them. "He was in his first coma last July," says Ned's mother. "It was a scary time, but we pulled through."

Pulling through is what people do around here. There is a kind of bravery in their lives that isn't bravery at all. It is automatic, unflinching, a mix of man and machine, consuming and unquestionable obligation meeting illness move for move in a giant, even-Steven game of chess: an unending round of something that looks like shadowboxing—though between love and death, which is the shadow? "Everyone admires us for our courage," says one man. "They have no idea what they're talking about."

I could get out of here, thinks the Mother. I could just get on a bus and go, never come back. Change my name. A kind of witness-relocation thing.

"Courage requires options," the man adds.

The Baby might be better off.

"There are options," says a woman with a thick suede headband. "You could give up. You could fall apart."

"No, you can't. Nobody does. I've never seen it," says the man. Well, not *really* fall apart." Then the lounge is quiet. Over the VCR someone has taped the fortune from a fortune cookie. *Optimism*, it says, *is what allows a teakettle to sing though up to its neck in hot water.* Underneath, someone else has taped a clipping from a summer horoscope. *Cancer rules!* it says. Who would tape this up? Somebody's twelve-year-old brother. One of the fathers—Joey's father—gets up and tears them both off, makes a small wad in his fist.

There is some rustling of magazine pages.

The Mother clears her throat. "Tiny Tim forgot the wet bar," she says.

Ned, who is still up, comes out of his room and down the corridor, whose lights dim at nine. Standing next to the Mother's chair, he says to her, "Where are you from? What is wrong with your baby?"

In the little room that is theirs, she sleeps fitfully in her sweatpants, occasionally leaping up to check on the Baby. This is what the sweatpants are for: leaping. In case of fire. In case of anything. In case the difference between day and night starts to dissolve and there is no difference at all so why pretend. In the cot beside her the Husband, who has taken a sleeping pill, is snoring loudly, his arms folded about his head in a kind of origami. How could either of them have stayed back at the house, with its empty high chair and empty crib? Occasionally the Baby wakes and cries out, and she bolts up, goes to him, rubs his back, rearranges the linens. The clock on the metal dresser shows that it is five after three. Then twenty to five. And then it is really morning, the beginning of this day, Nephrectomy Day. Will she be glad when it's over, or barely alive, or both? Each day of this week has arrived huge, empty, and unknown, like a spaceship, and this one especially is lit an incandescent gray.

"He'll need to put this on," says John, one of the nurses, bright and early, handing the Mother a thin greenish garment with roses and Teddy bears printed on it. A wave of nausea hits her: this smock, she thinks, will soon be splattered with—with what?

The Baby is awake but drowsy. She lifts off his pajamas. "Don't forget, *bubeleh*," she whispers, undressing and dressing him. "We will be with you every moment, every step. When you think you are asleep and floating off far away from everybody, Mommy will still be there." If she hasn't fled on a bus. "Mommy will take care of you. And Daddy, too." She hopes the Baby does not detect her own fear and uncertainty, which she must hide from him, like a limp. He is hungry, not having been allowed to eat, and he is no longer amused by this new place but worried about its hardships. Oh, my baby, she thinks. And the room starts to swim a little. The Husband comes in to take over. "Take a break," he says to her. "I'll walk him around for five minutes."

She leaves but doesn't know where to go. In the hallway she is approached by a kind of social worker, a customer-relations person, who had given them a video to watch about the anesthesia: how the parent accompanies the child into the operating room, and how gently, nicely the drugs are administered.

"Did you watch the video?"

"Yes," says the Mother.

"Wasn't it helpful?"

"I don't know," says the Mother.

"Do you have any questions?" asks the video woman. *Do you have any questions?* asked of someone who has recently landed in this fearful, alien place seems to the Mother an absurd and amazing little courtesy. The very specificity of a question would give the lie to the overwhelming strangeness of everything around her.

"Not right now," says the Mother. "Right now I think I'm just going to go to the bathroom."

When she comes back to the Baby's room, everyone is there: the Surgeon, the Anesthesiologist, all the nurses, the social worker. In their blue caps and scrubs they look like a clutch of forget-me-nots, and forget them who could? The Baby, in his little Teddy-bear smock, seems cold and scared. He reaches out and the Mother lifts him from the Husband's arms, rubs his back to warm him.

"Well, it's time!" says the Surgeon, forcing a smile.

"Shall we go?" says the Anesthesiologist.

What follows is a blur of obedience and bright lights. They take an elevator down to a big concrete room, the ante-room, the greenroom, the backstage of the operating room. Lining the walls are long shelves full of blue surgical outfits. "Children often become afraid of the color blue," one of the nurses says. But of course. Of course! "Now, which one of you would like to come into the operating room for the anesthesia?"

"I will," says the Mother.

"Are you sure?" says the Husband.

"Yup." She kisses the Baby's hair. Mr. Curlyhead people keep calling him here, and it seems both rude and nice. Women look admiringly at his long lashes and exclaim, "Always the boys! Always the boys!"

Two surgical nurses put a blue smock and a blue cotton cap on the Mother. The Baby finds this funny and keeps pulling at the cap. "This way," says another nurse, and the Mother follows. "Just put the Baby down on the table."

In the video, the mother holds the baby and fumes from the mask are gently waved under the baby's nose until he falls asleep. Now, out of view of camera or social worker, the Anesthesiologist is anxious to get this under way and not let too much gas leak out into the room generally. The occupational hazard of this, his chosen profession, is gas exposure and nerve damage, and it has started to worry him. No doubt he frets about it to his wife every night. Now he turns the gas on and quickly clamps the plastic mouthpiece over the Baby's cheeks and lips.

The Baby is startled. The Mother is startled. The Baby starts to scream and redden behind the plastic, but he cannot be heard. He thrashes. "Tell him it's O.K." says the nurse to the Mother.

O.K.? "It's O.K.," repeats the Mother, holding his hand, but she knows he can tell it's not O.K., because he can see that not only is she still wearing that stupid paper cap but her words are mechanical and swallowed, and she is biting her lips to keep them from trembling. Panicked, he attempts to sit, he cannot breathe, his arms reach up. *Bye-bye, outside.* And then, quite quickly, his eyes shut, he untenses and has fallen not into sleep but aside to sleep, an odd, kidnapping kind of sleep, his terror now hidden someplace deep inside him.

"How did it go?" asks the social worker, waiting in the concrete outer room. The Mother is hysterical. A nurse has ushered her out.

"It wasn't at all like the film strip!" she cries. "It wasn't like the film strip at all!"

"The film strip? You mean the video?" asks the social worker.

"It wasn't like that at all! It was brutal and unforgivable."

"Why, that's terrible," she says, her role now no longer misinformational but janitorial, and she touches the Mother's arm. The Mother shakes her off and goes to find the Husband.

She finds him in the large mulberry Surgery Lounge, where he has been taken and where there is free hot chocolate in small plastic-foam cups. Red cellophane garlands festoon the doorways. She has totally forgotten it is as close to Christmas as this. A pianist in the corner is playing "Carol of the Bells," and it sounds not only unfestive but scary, like the theme from "The Exorcist."

There is a giant clock on the far wall. It is a kind of porthole into the operating room, a way of assessing the Baby's ordeal: forty-five minutes for the Hickman implant; two and a half hours for the nephrectomy. And then, after that, three months of chemotherapy. The magazine on her lap stays open at a ruby-hued perfume ad.

"Still not taking notes," says the Husband.

"Nope."

"You know, in a way, this is the kind of thing you've *always* written about."

"You are really something, you know that? This is life. This isn't a 'kind of thing.'"

"But this is the kind of thing that fiction is: it's the unlivable life, the strange room tacked on to the house, the extra moon that is circling the earth unbeknownst to science."

"I told you that."

"I'm quoting you."

She looks at her watch, thinking of the Baby. "How long has it been?"

"Not long. Too long. In the end, those're the same things."

"What do you suppose is happening to him right this second?"

Infection? Slipping knives? "I don't know. But you know what? I've gotta go. I've gotta just walk a bit." The Husband gets up, walks around the lounge, then comes back and sits down.

The synapses between the minutes are unswimmable. An hour is thick as fudge. The Mother feels depleted; she is a string of empty tin cans attached by wire, something a goat would sniff and chew, something now and then enlivened by a jolt of electricity.

She hears their names being called over the intercom. "Yes? Yes?" She stands up quickly. Her voice has flown out before her, an exhalation of birds. The piano music has stopped. The pianist is gone. She and the Husband approach the main desk, where a man looks up at them and smiles. Before him is a Xeroxed list of patients' names. "That's our little boy right there," says the Mother, seeing the Baby's name on the list and pointing at it. "Is there some word? Is everything O.K.?"

"Yes," says the man. "Your boy is doing fine. They've just finished with the catheter and they are moving on to the kidney."

"But it's been two hours already! Oh, my God, did something go wrong, what happened, what went wrong?"

"Did something go wrong?" The Husband tugs at his collar.

"Not really. It just took longer than they expected. I'm told everything is fine. They wanted you to know."

"Thank you," says the Husband. They turn and walk back toward where they were sitting.

"I'm not going to make it," sighs the Mother, sinking into a fake-leather chair shaped somewhat like a baseball mitt. "But before I go I'm taking half this hospital out with me."

"Do you want some coffee?" asks the Husband.

"I don't know," says the Mother. "No, I guess not. No. Do you?"

"Nah, I don't, either, I guess," he says.

"Would you like part of an orange?"

"Oh, maybe, I guess, if you're having one." She takes a temple orange from her purse and just sits there peeling its difficult skin, the flesh rupturing beneath her fingers, the juice trickling down her hands, stinging the hangnails. She and the Husband chew and swallow, discreetly spit the seeds into Kleenex, and read from photocopies of the latest medical research which they begged from the interne. They read, and underline, and sigh and close their eyes, and after some time the surgery is over. A nurse from Peed-Onk comes down to tell them.

"Your little boy's in recovery right now. He's doing well. You can see him in about fifteen minutes."

How can it be described? How can any of it be described? The trip and the story of the trip are always two different things. The narrator is the one who has stayed home but then, afterward, presses her mouth upon the traveller's mouth, in order to make the mouth work, to make the mouth say, say, say. One cannot go to a place and speak of it, one cannot both see and say, not really. One can go, and upon returning make a lot of hand motions and indications with the arms. The mouth itself, working at the speed of light, at the eye's instructions, is necessarily struck still; so fast, so much to report, it hangs open and dumb as a gutted bell. All that unsayable life! That's where the narrator comes in. The narrator comes with her kisses and mimicry and tidying up. The narrator comes and makes a slow, fake song of the mouth's eager devastation.

It is a horror and a miracle to see him. He is lying in his crib in his room, tubed up, splayed like a boy on a cross, his arms stiffened into cardboard "no-no's" so that he cannot yank out the tubes. There is the bladder catheter, the nasal-gastric tube, and the Hickman, which, beneath the skin, is plugged into his jugular, then popped out his chest wall and capped with a long plastic cap. There is a large bandage taped over his abdomen. Groggy, on a morphine drip, still he is able to look at her when, maneuvering through all the vinyl wiring, she leans to hold him, and when she does he begins to cry, but cry silently, without motion or noise. She has never seen a baby cry without motion or noise. It is the crying of an old person: silent, beyond opinion, shattered. In someone so tiny, it is frightening and unnatural. She wants to pick up the Baby and run—out of there, out of there. She wants to whip out a gun: *No-no's, eh? This whole thing is what I call a no-no.* "Don't you touch him!" she wants to shout at the surgeons and the needle nurses. "Not anymore! No more! No more!" She would crawl up and lie beside him in the crib if she could. But instead, because of all his intricate wiring, she must lean and cuddle, sing to him, songs of peril and flight: "We gotta get out of this place, if it's the last thing we ever do. We gotta get out of this place. Baby, there's a better life for me and for you."

Very 1967. She was eleven then, and impressionable.

The Baby looks at her, pleadingly, his arms outstretched in surrender. To where? Where is there to go? Take me! Take me!

That night, post-op night, the Mother and the Husband lie afloat in their cots. A fluorescent lamp near the crib is kept on in the dark. The Baby breathes evenly but thinly in his drugged sleep. The morphine in its first flooding doses apparently makes him feel as if he were falling backward— or so the Mother has been told—and it causes the Baby to jerk, to catch himself over and over, as if he were being dropped from a tree. "Is this right? Isn't there something that should be done?" The nurses come in hourly, different ones—the night shifts seem strangely short and frequent. If the Baby stirs or frets, the nurses give him more morphine through the Hickman catheter, then leave to tend to other patients. The Mother rises to check on him herself in the low light. There is gurgling from the clear plastic suction tube coming out of his mouth. Brownish clumps have collected in the tube. What is going on? The Mother rings for the nurse. Is it Renee or Sarah or Darcy? She's forgotten.

"What, what is it?" murmurs the Husband, waking up.

"Something is wrong," says the Mother. "It looks like blood in his N-G tube."

"What?" The Husband gets out of bed. He, too, is wearing sweatpants.

The nurse—Valerie—pushes open the heavy door to the room and enters quietly. "Everything O.K.?"

"There's something wrong here. The tube is sucking blood out of his stomach. It looks like it may have perforated his stomach and now he's bleeding internally. Look!"

Valerie is a saint, but her voice is the standard hospital saint voice: an infuriating, pharmaceutical calm. It says, *Everything is normal here. Death is normal. Pain is normal. Nothing is abnormal. So there is nothing to get excited about.* "Well, now, let's see." She holds up the plastic tube and tries to see inside it. "Hmm," she says. "I'll call the attending physician."

Because this is a research and teaching hospital, all the regular doctors are at home sleeping in their Mission-style beds. Tonight, as is apparently the case every weekend night, the attending physician is a medical student. He looks fifteen: The authority he attempts to convey he cannot remotely inhabit. He is not even in the same building with it. He shakes everyone's hand, then strokes his chin, a gesture no doubt gleaned from some piece of dinner theatre his parents took him to once. As if there were an actual beard on that chin! As if beard growth on that chin were even possible! "Our Town"! "Kiss Me Kate"! "Barefoot in the Park"! He is attempting to convince if not to impress.

"We're in trouble," the Mother whispers to the Husband. She is tired, tired of young people grubbing for grades. "We've got Dr. 'Kiss Me Kate' here."

The Husband looks at her blankly, a mixture of disorientation and divorce.

The medical student holds the tubing in his hands. "I don't really see anything," he says.

He flunks! "You don't?" The Mother shoves her way in, holds the clear tubing in both hands. "That," she says. "Right here and here." Just this past semester she said to one of her own students, "If you don't see how this essay is better than that one, then I want you to just go out into the hallway and stand there until you do." Is it important to keep one's voice down? The Baby stays asleep. He is drugged and dreaming, far away.

"Hmm," says the medical student. "Perhaps there's a little irritation in the stomach."

"A little irritation?" The Mother grows furious. "This is blood. These are clumps and clots. This stupid thing is sucking the life right out of him!" Life! She is starting to cry.

They turn off the suction and bring in antacids, which they feed into the Baby through the tube. Then they turn the suction on again. This time on "low."

"What was it on before?" asks the Husband.

"High," says Valerie. "Doctor's orders, though I don't know why. I don't know why these doctors do a lot of the things they do."

"Maybe they're—not all that bright?" suggests the Mother. She is feeling relief and rage simultaneously: there is a feeling of prayer and litigation in the air. Yet essentially she is grateful. Isn't she? She thinks she is. And still, and still: look at all the things you have to do to protect a child, a hospital merely an intensification of life's cruel obstacle course.

The Surgeon comes to visit on Saturday morning. He steps in and nods at the Baby, who is awake but glazed from the morphine, his eyes two dark, unseeing grapes. "The boy looks fine," he announces. He peeks under the Baby's bandage. "The stitches look good," he says. The Baby's abdomen is stitched all the way across, like a baseball. "And the other kidney, when we looked at it yesterday face to face, looked fine. We'll try to wean him off the morphine a little, and see how he's doing on Monday."

"Is he going to be O.K.?"

"The boy? The boy is going to be fine," he says, then taps her stiffly on the shoulder. "Now, you take care. It's Saturday. Drink a little wine."

Over the weekend, while the Baby sleeps, the Mother and the Husband sit together in the Tiny Tim Lounge. The Husband is restless and makes cafeteria and sundry runs, running errands for everyone. In his absence, the other parents regale her further with their sagas. Pediatric cancer and chemo stories: the children's amputations, blood poisoning, teeth flaking like shale, the learning delays and disabilities caused by chemo frying the young, budding brain. But strangely optimistic codas are tacked on: endings as stiff and loopy as carpenter's lace, crisp and empty as lettuce, reticulate as a net—ah, words. "After all that business with the tutor, he's better now, and fitted with new incisors by my wife's cousin's husband, who did dental school in two and a half years, if you can believe that. We hope for the best. We take things as they come. Life is hard."

"Life's a big problem," agrees the Mother. Part of her welcomes and invites all their tales. In the few long days since this nightmare began, part of her has become addicted to disaster and war stories. She only wants to hear about the sadness and emergencies of others. They are the only situations that can join hands with her own; everything else bounces off her shiny shield of resentment and unsympathy. Nothing else can even stay in her brain. From this, no doubt, the philistine world is made, or should one say recruited? Together the parents huddle all day in the Tiny Tim Lounge—no need to watch "Oprah." They leave Oprah in the dust. Oprah has nothing on them. They chat matter-of-factly, then fall silent and watch "Dune" or "Star Wars," in which there are bright and shiny robots, whom the Mother now sees not as robots at all but as human beings who have had terrible things happen to them.

Some of their friends visit with stuffed animals and soft "Looking good"s for the dozing baby, though the room is way past the stuffed-animal limit. The Mother arranges, once more, a plateful of Mint Milano cookies and cups of takeout coffee for guests. All her nutso pals stop by—the two on Prozac, the one obsessed with the word "penis" in the word "happiness," the one who recently had her hair foiled green. "Your friends put the *de* in *fin de siècle*," says the Husband. Overheard, or recorded, all marital conversation sounds as if someone must be joking, though usually no one is.

She loves her friends, especially loves them for coming, since there are times they all fight and don't speak for weeks. Is this friendship? For now and here, it must do and is, and is, she swears it is. For one, they never offer impromptu spiritual lectures about death, how it is part of life, its natural ebb and flow, how we all must accept that, or other such utterances that make her want to scratch out somebody's eyes. Like true friends, they take no hardy or elegant stance loosely choreographed from some broad perspective. They get right in there and mutter "Jesus Christ!" and shake their heads. Plus, they are the only people who will not only laugh at her stupid jokes but offer up stupid ones of their own. *What do you get when you cross Tiny Tim with a pit bull?* A child's illness is a strain on the mind. They know how to laugh in a flutey, desperate way—unlike the people who are more her husband's friends and who seem just to deepen their sorrowful gazes, nodding their heads in Sympathy. How Exiling and Estranging are everybody's Sympathetic Expressions! When anyone laughs, she thinks, O.K. Hooray! A buddy. In disaster as in show business.

Nurses come and go; their chirpy voices both startle and soothe. Some of the other Peed-Onk parents stick their heads in to see how the Baby is and offer encouragement.

Green Hair scratches her head: "Everyone's so friendly here. Is there someone in this place who isn't doing all this airy, scripted optimism—or are people like that the only people here?"

"It's Modern Middle Medicine meets the Modern Middle Family," says the Husband. "In the Modern Middle West."

Someone has brought in takeout lo mein, and they all eat it out in the hall by the elevators.

Parents are allowed use of the Courtesy Line.

"You've got to have a second child," says a friend on the phone, a friend from out of town. "An heir and a spare. That's what we did. We had another child to insure we wouldn't off ourselves if we lost our first."

"Really?"

"I'm serious."

"A formal suicide? Wouldn't you just drink yourself into a lifelong stupor and let it go at that?"

"Nope. I knew how I would do it even. For a while, until our second came along, I had it all planned."

"You did? What did you plan?"

"I can't go into too much detail, because—hi, honey!—the kids are here now in the room. But I'll spell out the general idea: R-O-P-E."

Sunday evening she goes and sinks down on the sofa in the Tiny Tim Lounge next to Frank, Joey's father. He is a short, stocky man with the currentless, flat-lined look behind the eyes that all the parents eventually get here. He has shaved his head bald in solidarity with his son. His little boy has been battling cancer for five years. It is now in the liver, and the rumor around the corridor is that Joey has three weeks to live. She knows that Joey's mother, Roseanne, left Frank years ago, two years into the cancer, and has remarried and had another child, a girl named Brittany. The Mother sees Roseanne here sometimes with her new life—the cute little girl and the new full-haired husband, who will never be so maniacally and debilitatingly obsessed with Joey's illness the way Frank, her first husband, is. Roseanne comes to visit Joey, to say hello and now goodbye, but she is not Joey's main man. Frank is.

Frank is full of stories—about the doctors, about the food, about the nurses, about Joey. Joey, affectless from his meds, sometimes leaves his room and comes out to watch TV in his bathrobe. He is jaundiced and bald, and though he is nine he looks no older than six. Frank has devoted the last four and a half years to saving Joey's life. When the cancer was first diagnosed, the doctors gave Joey a twenty-per-cent chance of living six more months. Now here it is almost five years later, and Joey's still here. It is all due to Frank, who, early on, quit his job as vice-president of a consulting firm in order to commit himself totally to his son. He is proud of everything he's given up and done, but he is tired. Part of him now really believes that things are coming to a close, that this is the end. He says this without tears. There are no more tears.

"You have probably been through more than anyone else on this corridor," says the Mother.

"I could tell you stories," he says. There is a sour odor between them, and she realizes that neither of them has bathed for days.

"Tell me one. Tell me the worst one." She knows he hates his ex-wife and hates her new husband even more.

"The worst? They're all the worst. Here's one: one morning I went out for breakfast with my buddy—it was the only time I'd left Joey alone ever, left him for two hours is all—and when I came back his N-G tube was full of blood. They had the suction on too high, and it was sucking the guts right out of him."

"Oh, my God. That just happened to us," said the Mother.

"It did?"

"Friday night."

"You're kidding. They let that happen again? I gave them such a chewing out about that!"

"I guess our luck is not so good. We get your very worst story on the second night we're here."

"It's not a bad place, though."

"It's not?"

"Naw. I've seen worse. I've taken Joey everywhere."

"He seems very strong." Truth is, at this point Joey seems like a zombie and frightens her.

"Joey's a fucking genius. A biological genius. They'd given him six months, remember."

The Mother nods.

"Six months is not very long," says Frank. "Six months is nothing. He was four and a half years old."

All the words are like blows. She feels flooded with affection and mourning for this man. She looks away, out the window, out past the hospital parking lot, up toward the black marbled sky and the electric eyelash of the moon. "And now he's nine," she says. "You're his hero."

"And he's mine," says Frank, though the fatigue in his voice seems to overwhelm him. "He'll be that forever. Excuse me," he says. "I've got to go check. His breathing hasn't been good. Excuse me."

"Good news and bad," says the Oncologist on Monday. He has knocked, entered the room, and now stands there. Their cots are unmade. One wastebasket is overflowing with coffee cups. "We've got the pathologist's report. The bad news is that the kidney they removed had certain lesions, called 'rests,' which are associated with a higher risk for disease in the other kidney. The good news is that the tumor is Stage I, regular cell structure, and under five hundred grams, which qualifies you for a national experiment in which chemotherapy isn't done but your boy is simply monitored with ultrasound. It's not all that risky, given that the patient's watched closely, but here is the literature on it. There are forms to sign, if you decide to do that. Read all this and we can discuss it further. You have to decide within four days."

Lesions? Rests? They dry up and scatter like M&M's on the floor. All she hears is the part about no chemo. Another sigh of relief rises up in her and spills out. In a life where there is only the bearable and the unbearable, a sigh of relief is an ecstasy.

"No chemo?" says the husband. "Do you recommend that?"

The Oncologist shrugs. What casual gestures these doctors are permitted! "I know chemo. I like chemo," says the Oncologist. "But this is for you to decide. It depends how you feel."

The Husband leans forward. "But don't you think that now that we have the upper hand with this thing we should keep going? Shouldn't we stomp on it, beat it, smash it to death with the chemo?"

The Mother swats him angrily and hard. "Honey, you're delirious!" She whispers, but it comes out as a hiss. "This is our lucky break." Then she adds gently, "We don't want the Baby to have chemo."

The Husband turns back to the Oncologist. "What do you think?"

"It could be," he says, shrugging. "It could be that this is your lucky break. But you won't know for sure for five years."

The Husband turns back to the Mother. "O.K.," he says. "O.K."

The Baby grows happier and strong. He begins to move and sit and eat. Wednesday morning they are allowed to leave, and to leave without chemo. The Oncologist looks a little nervous. "Are you nervous about this?" asks the Mother.

"Of course I'm nervous." But he shrugs and doesn't look that nervous.

"See you in six weeks for the ultrasound," he says, then he waves and leaves, looking at his big black shoes.

The Baby smiles, even toddles around a little, the sun bursting through the clouds, an angel chorus crescendoing. Nurses arrive. The Hickman is taken out of the Baby's neck and chest, antibiotic lotion is dispensed. The Mother packs up their bags. The baby sucks on a bottle of juice and does not cry.

"No chemo?" says one of the nurses. "Not even a little chemo?"

"We're doing watch-and-wait," says the Mother.

The other parents look envious but concerned. They have never seen any child get out of there with his hair and white blood cells intact.

"Will you be O.K.?" says Ned's mother.

"The worry's going to kill us," says the Husband.

"But if all we have to do is worry," chides the Mother, "every day for a hundred years, it'll be easy. It'll be nothing. I'll take all the worry in the world if it wards off the thing itself."

"That's right," says Ned's mother. "Compared to everything else, compared to all the actual events, the worry is nothing."

The Husband shakes his head. "I'm such an amateur," he moans.

"You're both doing admirably," says the other mother. "Your baby's lucky, and I wish you all the best."

The Husband shakes her hand warmly. "Thank you," he says. "You've been wonderful."

Another mother, the mother of Eric, comes up to them. "It's all very hard," she says, her head cocked to one side. "But there's a lot of collateral beauty along the way."

Collateral beauty? Who is entitled to such a thing? A child is ill. No one is entitled to any collateral beauty.

"Thank you," says the Husband.

Joey's father, Frank, comes up and embraces them both. "It's a journey," he says. He chucks the Baby on the chin. "Good luck, little man."

"Yes, thank you so much," says the Mother. "We hope things go well with Joey." She knows that Joey had a hard, terrible night.

Frank shrugs and steps back "Gotta go," he says. "Goodbye!"

"Bye," she says, and then he is gone. She bites the inside of her lip, a bit tearily, then bends down to pick up the diaper bag, which is now stuffed with little animals; helium balloons are tied to its zipper. Shouldering the thing, the Mother feels she has just won a prize. All the parents have now vanished down the hall in the opposite direction. The Husband moves close. With one arm he takes the Baby from her; with the other he rubs her back. He can see she is starting to get weepy.

"Aren't these people nice? Don't you feel better hearing about their lives?" he asks.

Why does he do this, form clubs all the time—why does even this society of suffering soothe him? When it comes to death and dying, perhaps someone in this family ought to be more of a snob.

"All these nice people with their brave stories," he continues as they make their way toward the elevator bank, waving goodbye to the nursing staff as they go, even the Baby waving shyly. *Bye-bye! Bye-bye!* "Don't you feel consoled, knowing we're all in the same boat, that we're all in this together?"

But who on earth would want to be in this boat? the Mother thinks. This boat is a nightmare boat. Look where it goes: to a silver-and-white room, where, just before your eyesight and hearing and your ability to touch or be touched disappear entirely, you must watch your child die.

Rope! Bring on the rope.

"Let's make our own way," says the Mother, "and not in this boat."

Woman Overboard! She takes the Baby back from the Husband, cups the Baby's cheek in her hand, kisses his brow and then, quickly, his flowery mouth. The Baby's heart—she can hear it—drums with life. "For as long as I live," says the Mother, pressing the elevator button—up or down, everyone in the end has to leave this way—"I never want to see any of these people again."

There are the notes.

Now, where is the money?

25

Children's Ward

❧ Sarah Day

In this room, a melancholy alliance
of breathlessness exists, a children's wind ensemble
hooting through the weary nocturne.

Here above the city, it's another world.
Like a pressurised aircraft at night
the hum insinuates itself into rows of dreams.

Despite the dimness, there is not enough light
to unhook the eyelids' high-tension wire
and dissolve into mind's darkness.

She has been stroking his back since time began,
working calm's liniment between shoulder blades
scarcely bigger than chicken wings.

I am awake. Breathing for her child in the corner,
trying not to think of landed fish, pop-eyed,
drowning in air. His panic mounts until

sweet as frangipani, his mother's dulcet voice
sings out an aria—
the two syllables of his name.

Between vertical slits of venetian light
nurses' talk drifts on long-distance radio waves.
Torchlight pads through the half sleep

disclosing parents camped on cots like refugees.
Eventually dawn will lighten into grey
behind double glaze.

Above the dull city, focus narrows
to the hand's circular motion.
Sleeping, the ear conch listens,

trained on the beat of a heart,
the strength of an indrawn breath.
As long as the hand strokes, and while the voice
croons . . .

26

Parents Support Group

✑ Dick Allen

Our children half-lost, we gather at the table,
Making small polite jokes
About weather and coffee. The blinds are drawn.
Outside, the summer afternoon is tennis strokes,

A grackle calling to its mate, wind-chimes
Sliding tailgates of delivery vans. Long-timers smile
And pat the new arrivals' backs. Our therapist
Takes a long, long, long, long, *long* while

Before he starts, reluctantly. That hot potato, Pain,
Goes round and round the table. Who of us
Are blameless, who share blame
For why our children left a crust

Of blood across their wrists, gulped pills, or think
Their terribly thin bodies still are fat,
Did drugs, did drink
Behind ripped billboards of their raw self-hate?

We don't know. Weeks . . . or was it days ago,
Self-tucked in the illusion we control
Our lives . . . sane, in our accepting this . . . we thought
That all stones roll

Downhill, all rabbits leap, the months ahead
Are simply spaces on our calendars
Where plans are penciled or not penciled in.
That's normal and not wrong . . . but now we're here

Talking with strangers. To our left
The lady in a green dress weeps; the man
Whose daughter must be begged or bribed to eat
Keeps putting up and putting down his hand,

Then polishing his glasses on his paisley tie.
I don't know what to say. I don't know anything
That can help us all. Words alone
(How many words there were!) have come unstrung

And scatter everywhere. Back in their halls
Our children hunch above their Scrabble board,
Or shoot the breeze
As aimlessly as they shot down our world.

27

Starter

⚬ *Amy Hanridge*

For Emily

Everybody says they joined the military because of 9-11. They wanted to be a hero, patriotic or what not. And who wouldn't? I was all for those things. I never had anything against any of that. But if I was honest, I'd tell people I signed with the Marine Corps because I couldn't see any reason not to. I don't tell anybody this, though.

I don't lie. They just don't ask. They assume it's because of 9-11 and I don't correct them.

And now that I'm out, sure there's a pride there that I served. I bump into old high school friends like Makayla Lupe at Le Nails or even my old boyfriend Emilius Alchesay at Video Dome and they go on about how they missed me. They heard I was back from Mama or my sister. They think our troops are doing a great job over there. They say, "Wow, I bet your niece is huge to you, born while you were deployed and all."

I just shrug, but my mind never goes to 9-11. It travels straight to the recruiter's office, down a narrow hallway with blue faux wood paneling—who ever heard of blue wood, anyway?—and the skinny man who leaned in too close as I signed my papers. Every enlistee's experience in a recruiter's office is different. I'm sure the kids right after 9-11 heard a lot about pride and doing what's right for your country, but I was a little too late for that talk, I suppose, or my recruiter just knew that approach doesn't work with Apaches. Lori Piestewa, that Hopi girl all over the news when she was killed in Iraq, already had a mountain named after her in Phoenix by the time I picked up my pen. Everybody was already over their shock and awe by then. I just knew I'd graduated far enough from the top of my class that scholarships were out of the question, so the Marines made sense.

I'm big like I remember Dad was, before he left us. Mama always described Dad, and now me, as "tall and intimidating." She said it made sense that I'd be a Marine. She said I look like one. Mama and my sister Lynneaya are both tiny.

While I was away, Mama got me a German Shepherd. I think she felt bad because she never got me a dog when I was a kid and always asked her for one. She taught it to sleep in a wire crate with the door open. The kennel is right next to my bed and as soon as I got back I had to feel guilty for sleeping all day because the dog never got any exercise. He'd just lie in his crate, waiting for me to wake up. I named him Gunny, after my gunnery sergeant. I saw Gunny on Skype when he was just a puppy and Mama held him up to her slow computer. He was huge by the time I got home.

Once I'd been home a while, Mama started asking me to see someone about my "difficulties," as she called them. She worried about me. I tried to get in to see a shrink at the VA and it's like ten years until I can get in to see one. Mama worried I'd do like Dad did if I waited too long to see a VA shrink. She talked to a friend of hers from Gadfly, the little ski town that borders our Apache reservation. Her friend is some white gal she works with, whose sister is a family therapist who gets all teary eyed about Jesus and the Veterans. The sister thinks all vets sacrificed themselves just for her. I guess the sister wanted to do something nice for a veteran. I got volunteered. She agreed to see me for free. Her office is in the same thin-walled building where the recruiter was all those years ago. Only her paneling is green fake wood instead of blue.

So, Judy Jones is the name of my shrink. She hates it when I call her a shrink. She's my "therapist." She doesn't say hate. I don't think she'd say she hates anything, except maybe people who forget Veterans. She's big on remembering us. When I call her my shrink, she tilts her head to one side and looks at me through the tops of her eyeglasses to correct me. "Therapist, Ms. Henry."

She always calls me Ms. Henry, too. In high school, I was always just Henry. More often than Kayla. Same with the military. Henry or Private Henry. Or Private. Never Miss, and never ever Ms.

I think I surprise Judy Jones because I will at least talk to her. She has the idea that all Apaches are mute. She watches too many reruns of cowboy and Indian movies on cable. Actually, I used to be a chatterbox. Mama says I would drive her crazy telling her everything I was thinking about all the time. What I ate, how it digested, who was mean, who was cute, what I thought about the wind. Mama says even as a little girl I would wake her up in the middle of the night and tell her how Mr. Wind was bugging me. She'd hand me a can of air freshener and tell me to scare Mr. Wind with it. That was the closest thing in her reach one night when all she wanted to do was go back to sleep and the idea stuck. After that, she'd come in to my room most mornings and there'd be a stinky fog that would just about knock her over and I'd be chattering right in the middle of it about how I'd tried and tried all night to frighten Mr. Wind away but he was still buggin' me.

I guess I don't talk near as much as I used to, though, and that's what's scaring Mama. That's why she wanted me to talk with Judy Jones. That and how I scared the baby. Judy Jones and I talk about this; she says I'll tell her about it when I'm ready.

Judy Jones asks me what kind of things I like to do. "Nothing much," I tell her. She doesn't believe me and presses me for an answer. Til one day I just told her: "I used to like going to the grocery store parking lot in town every day for lunch." I told her how everybody called it the Rez Café, though it was only a line of tents and card tables at the back of the parking lot. The grocery manager still lets the old ladies set up there because they buy their flour and salt in the store. I used to pick a different fry bread stand depending on the day. Rudy Altaha's on Mondays, because she always pressure-cooked her beans so they were the creamiest and that somehow made Monday more bearable. Lois Naseyoma's on Tuesdays because she always used greens from her own garden shredded on top. Curtis Crier's on Wednesday because he never used fresh veggies any other day but got them fresh from the farmer's market every Wednesday. Oh, and never Frederica Lupe's stand. Just never. She reused her oil a thousand times and it always tasted like mothballs.

Judy Jones asked me have I been back to the Rez Café lately. I told her I went for lunch since I've been back, and tried to eat an Apache taco, from Rudy Altaha even—she's still there in her camp dress, crinkling her eyes and flashing her tooth for every customer—but somehow even her beans don't taste as smooth as they used to. Maybe she skips the lard nowadays. Everybody's quitting the lard because it's bad for the heart. But things don't taste the same without it.

Mama came into my room the other morning and told me she's been praying to God that I'll start liking the things I used to like and that I'll find something to do for myself. Later, that night, we were at the dinner table. Lynneaya took the baby in the stroller to go walk around the lake, so it was just Mama and me, eating hamburger steak and peas. Mama asked me what I was thinking. I told her she didn't want to know what I was thinking, but she pushed me like Judy Jones does. So I said, "You used to pray for me every day, Mama. You told me in every email, every phone call, every care package." I tossed some peas around on my plate with my fork. "Maybe I still need that."

Mama said, "You think I don't?"

I put down my fork.

"I pray for you even more now," she said, "because I can tell I need to."

She stood up and carried her plate to the kitchen. She came back for salt and pepper, talking like she never left the room. "But I haven't told you, because I haven't wanted to make you feel bad." The salt and pepper shakers knocked together as she took them in one hand while pulling my plate away with her other hand. I hadn't touched my meat or my peas, but I guess she could tell I was finished.

"If it's God's will," she said. "I told God I wanted you back to your old self, only if it was His will." She headed back into the kitchen and said over her shoulder, "I also told him, if he'd like to hear my opinion on things, then my opinion is I hope my daughter is her old self."

I guess Mama started really worrying about me after I first got home and Mama and Lynneaya left me alone with the baby one day. Lynneaya got called into work. A bunch of tour buses filled with old people from California rolled into the casino parking lot and I remember Lynneaya saying her boss wanted "all hands on deck." I wondered if the boss even knew what that really meant. I remember Mama asking Lynneaya what she was going to do with the baby. Lynneaya walked out the screen door and hollered on the way to her car, "Let Kayla do it. She's home all day."

Mama came up to me and put her hands on my shoulders, shaking me a little. "You have to help us out here." Then it was just me and the baby. The crib is in the living room next to the TV. For the longest time I sat in the recliner across the room, watching the baby's belly go up and down. It was on its back and its arms were up and over its head and its legs were wide apart. It looked like a little "x" just flopped there on the mattress with nothing but a cream-colored fitted sheet on it. I shocked myself a bit when I peeked at her through the bars and said, "Splat" out loud. That's what she looked like, like she'd just fallen from somewhere, splat, right onto the pad.

That is, until she woke up. She was silent for so long, just the up and down of her belly through her tight yellow t-shirt, then all of a sudden she sucked in a big gasp of air and she sat up. She took one look at me across the room and another quick scan to see Lynneaya and Mama were gone, and she started up with hiccup cries, followed right after with full-on screams. I flapped around the house a while, finding blankies and bottles. I washed off a pacifier I found on the kitchen floor.

The baby wanted none of it. She wanted none of me. She kept leaning past me, craning to see into the kitchen or the other side into Mama's bedroom, probably hoping they'd walk in and save her from me. The whole time she just kept screaming, louder and louder.

That's when I felt myself starting to get mad. Hadn't I done what Mama and Lynneaya would have done? I turned my back on the baby, walked to the kitchen, around to the bathroom, back through Mama's bedroom and into the living room again. I put my hands on my low back.

There was still the screaming. Except now, was it just the baby doing the screaming? Next thing I knew, my hands weren't on my low back, but the baby's. I was lifting her up, out of the crib. I was the one screaming. I was shaking her, toward me and away. "Snap out of it!" Those were my words. "Snap out of it! Stop being such a baby!"

That's when Mama walked in on us. "Kayla!" she said, and she elbowed me in the stomach as she pulled the baby out of my arms.

So, yeah, Mama made me start seeing Judy Jones. The baby's okay, but I don't want to think about what might have happened had Mama not come home for lunch.

Judy Jones wants me to talk about things like this. Therapy still doesn't make much sense to me, but I do what Judy Jones says. Especially when I'm late for an appointment or I try to skip and she calls me or finds me at Coffee Chalet and growls in a low voice, "Get to my office. Now." She reminds me of my Staff Sergeant when she does that. I snap to and do what she says. I start spilling whatever comes to me.

Like, just the other day I got to thinking, I don't know why this popped into my brain, but I told it to Judy Jones, about Mama's starter bread. Mama doesn't make it anymore. She doesn't even make fry bread anymore. Everybody's so busy. I think Mama has a jar of it in the bottom of the freezer, but she doesn't make homemade bread everyday like she used to, grinding her own wheat and using nothing but that, some water, salt and the starter that our family's had around for who-knows-how-long, first collected from the white powder on juniper berries. I got to thinking about that quart jar Mama always kept in the fridge. She had to bake bread all the time just to keep the juniper starter alive. It was right about the time Daddy left, and Mama forgot to put the lid on gentle. She used to lecture to me, Don't put the lid on tight, but I never knew why. Mama must have been distracted by Daddy leaving because she screwed the lid on tight and forgot about that jar.

I opened up the fridge one day to get some milk, I was always drinking milk those days, and there were shards of glass and globs of alcohol-smelling flour all over the refrigerator. Mama came home, dropped to her knees and cried. She had named her starter Monster, like it was a pet that lived in our fridge. And now it was gone. DesiMae Altaha brought us over a jar of her starter the next day, because she knew how sad Mama was. But Mama said it wasn't from her family so it wasn't the same.

I don't know what made me think of those shards of glass all of a sudden. I guess I saw some broken glass reflecting sun on the side of the road while I was out walking and thought of that explosion. I miss that bread. Mama always made the best bread.

Judy Jones asks me questions sometimes, especially when I'm quiet and don't know what to talk about. She says I need to talk about what's on my mind. Sometimes I don't know what's on my mind, only that I'm tired all the time. I can't sleep. As soon as my head nods, if I'm in the big brown chair in the living room, I startle. As soon as I'm quiet and start to fall asleep in bed, my body jerks and I let out an "Ah!"

Not too long ago Judy Jones asked me, "How were you treated as a woman in the military?"

All I said was, "I had to keep up." I was in no mood.

"Yes," she said. She wasn't giving up. She sat forward in her black leather chair. She touched her fingertips together and she held her shoulders up high. I've noticed how she pushes me when her shoulders are hiked up, like she's trying to convince me of something. ". . . But how were you treated, you know, personally, back in the barracks?"

I flopped farther back in my seat and dug my shoe into her rug. "Look, this isn't going to be an Oprah show or some women's group."

Judy Jones looked surprised.

"God, you remind me of a teacher I had in junior high health class. She wore dangle earrings and scarves every single day. It was a class just for us girls and, besides the birds and the bees, the teacher was always trying to get us to spill our feelings about how we were 'treated.' Who does that?"

She looked at me over those eyeglasses and said, "What's your point, Ms. Henry?" Her voice was quiet and her shoulders were down again.

I sat up and looked around the room. Good question. I thought about it for a long while and said, "I loved the military, that's all."

Judy Jones saw this as her opening to use her therapist voice. She uses it every once in a while—her slow, pointed voice, sounds like the bishop at Mama's church. He pauses for effect and makes a big deal. She'd get my attention better if she'd use her Staff Sergeant growl. Instead she breathed out, "You can love it and it can still hurt you."

I stood up. I had to move. I felt myself grinding my teeth as I walked around her room. I said, "Aw, hell. There are a lot of complainers that seem to crawl out of the woodwork once they leave the military. There are probably complainers everywhere. You won't catch me being one of them."

Judy Jones took one more opportunity that day to use Therapist Voice: "Needing help doesn't make you a complainer." She must have caught on that her tone was getting to me because quick as she turned it on, she just dropped it and said normally, "Group therapy would help you, if we can find people like you who have gone through experiences like yours."

Hearing her drop something and just talk to me regular made me drop my act, too. I sat down next to her again and asked, "Who is like me, really? How many Apache women soldiers do you know?"

She said, "Don't kid yourself, Ms. Henry. Don't get to thinking you're

all alone. That's dangerous thinking. First and foremost, we are human animals. We invented speech as a species for a reason. We may not be able to
get our points across perfectly. We may not be able to get people to understand us completely, but we should never give up trying. That's what speech
is for. We communicate. We keep talking. We keep trying. To do any less is
to literally deny our own humanity. That's the greatest risk of all."

Judy Jones is like a boxer in the way she gets me to talk about my de-
ployment. She dances, then jabs. She starts talking about my favorite food,
then what I missed over there, then—bam!—we're in Iraq and she's asking
me what my job was like. I'm not afraid to talk about it. Most days what I
did was typical, but I guess there was always the potential for more because
I patted down injured Iraqi women before they were admitted to the E.R. I
was trained to find bombs on them, just most times I didn't.

So one day Judy Jones is doing her dance and jab routine when she
throws me an uppercut. She asks me full on about the time I did find a
bomb on a woman. Only it wasn't a woman, it was a girl. What's worse, she
was one of the Iraqi children I knew. I recognized her right off.

Those kinds of things happened over there. We used to go out and give
gum and candy to the neighborhood kids. We were only cleared to do this
when we were supported and only then in the secured area, but I got used
to seeing this one girl. I'd remember her because instead of the one word in
English all the other kids knew, "Candy," she'd holler, "One pen." Just like
that. "One pen." Not just "pen." Somebody had taught her to say "one pen,"
and after a while I brought a ballpoint, just to see if she really wanted it.

I will always remember how excited she was. I can't describe her eyes.
She was like a flower opening. Sure enough, all she wanted was a pen.

When they brought her in to the E.R. on the gurney, her whole left side
was bleeding. She was awake and looked at me. I don't know if she recognized me. The flower look in her eyes was gone. It didn't take me long to
find the bomb material taped to her back side. With the girl in her draping
black dress, it could have easily gone unnoticed and killed who knows and
how many inside the hospital.

Judy Jones asked me if I felt betrayed. I must have snorted or let out one
of my harrumphs because she took offense at my response.

"Ms. Henry," she said, "if you don't want to talk, fine. Let's call it a day.
But don't you dare disrespect me."

"I wasn't trying to disrespect you, Ma'am," I said.

"You might not have been trying, but you succeeded."

"No, Ma'am," I said. "It was the word 'betrayed.' You asked me if I felt
betrayed."

"Yes, and you scoffed at me," Judy Jones said.

"That scoff wasn't at you, Ma'am. It was at my own mind, I guess."

"What do you mean?"

I tried to explain how ironic it was that I've never felt betrayed by the girl with the bomb, someone who could have killed me. I mean, to this day I don't know if she willingly put that bomb on herself or if someone made her, but either way I don't care.

"What is ironic, Ms. Henry?"

"There's only one person who I'd ever say betrayed me and it's not the person who might have killed me with a bomb," I said.

"Who is it, then?"

"Joe."

"Who is Joe?"

"My boyfriend."

That seemed to turn something on inside Judy Jones. She exploded with questions about Joe: When did we meet? Was it in the military? Were we deployed together? I interrupted her with, "Look, if anything, the military was a coincidence in our relationship; it was certainly a coincidence in our breakup and I don't want to talk about it."

That choked off our conversation for that day. She ended with, "I won't make you talk about Joe, but you should talk about him with someone. Perhaps your mother."

We went along in that strangled way in our sessions for a while. I started trying to skip appointments again and Judy Jones took to yanking me out of The Bear's Den Bar to bring me to her office. Until she asked me the other day, "What's the main thing you learned while you were over there?"

I surprised myself by having an answer right away.

I told her that the main thing I learned in Iraq is I'm not special. We're not special. Nobody's special. Growing up, Mama made me feel we were different, important, mostly because we went to church. We made the right choices, were closer to God somehow. But over there I realized, there are six billion of us. Six billion of God's "chosen" people.

I also realized, we're all kidding ourselves. Over there, you could be the most decorated soldier, the smartest one, the one who followed all the rules and humped the fastest and worked the hardest and carried the most gear and you could still get blown to Kingdom Come by a roadside bomb. That's what happened to chosen people.

The bomb knew the truth. The bomb knew there wasn't a one of us was special. We were all just bait for the bomb. I suppose that girl with the bomb strapped to her, the one I gave the pen to, she probably believed she was special. Somebody probably told her there'd be a special place in heaven for her. Or people who believed there was a special place in heaven for them made her wear that bomb. I suppose I should have hated her, or the people who made her do it. Maybe I should have wanted to rip them all to pieces for trying to blow me up with her. But if I felt that, it'd mean I cared, or that I believed I was the one who was right, and she was the one who was wrong. Only I don't believe that. I have so much distance from all that. I just shake my head and think the poor girl thinks she matters. What a fool.

After I said all this to Judy Jones, she said to me, "You can be ordinary, Ms. Henry. You can be one of six billion, and you can still matter."

I think I did my harrumph thing and she got on me for brushing her off again. Then she said, "It's like your mom's starter you told me about."

I lifted my head her way. She had my attention because she was telling my stories back to me.

"You said your mom didn't want her friend's starter because it wasn't the same." Judy Jones raised her shoulders to her ears again. She was on a roll. "Someone in your family collected wild yeast off of juniper berries, cultured it, preserved it and passed it on." Her eyebrows were up and she was nodding her head up and down like she wanted me to agree with her. I just sat there.

"Don't you know, Ms. Henry? Your mom's right. Her friend's mixture wouldn't have been the same." She looked at me over the tops of her glasses again. "You are the starter, Ms. Henry. And so am I. And so is everybody. There may be other ways to bake bread in the world, from juniper berries, from grapes, from a plastic bag in a grocery store, but none of it would be the same as yours. You can be one of six billion and you can still matter." Judy Jones danced and jabbed my story right back at me.

I get tired of all the emails in my in box that try to make me pay attention by telling me these are the type of stories you'll never hear. That's what I said to Judy Jones recently. Why do they have to dress up the stories that way, I asked her. Who cares whether you'll ever hear these stories or not? Stories deserve to be told, that's all. Why can't they just say that? And even if you hear the same story over and over again, that doesn't make it less important. Just tell the stories. I guess I'm starting to listen to what Judy Jones is teaching me.

Folks in the military are heroes, every day. And folks in the military are ordinary, just like me. We get in bad moods, do stupid things, selfish things. We also do generous things and once in a while we get things right. We do a job that requires us to get our affairs in order before we even start it, that's all. I remember the day Mama called me on my cell, crying, when the mail came with my Last Will and Testament and my plans for who would get my personal effects if I died in Iraq. She didn't make any sense.

She blubbered and the only word I could make out was "Don't." I never wanted to do that to Mama. I didn't want to think about that stuff myself, but you do it. It's your job. It's part of the mission.

It reminds me of the time we were evacuated because of the Paradise Creek Fire. At the time, it was the biggest forest fire Arizona had ever seen. Bunches of us stayed in our tents at the rodeo grounds. Reporters were there from all over, shoving their microphones into our faces and zooming their video cameras up close. They asked us how it felt to have our whole community at risk of being burned up. All I remember thinking is I don't want to be this person on the news. I don't want to be the person folks shake their head at while they're eating their supper in front of the TV, tsk-tsking and moaning, "What a shame" or "Those poor people." I didn't want to be the person people felt bad about. I still don't. I just want to live my life.

I felt that way in the military and I feel that way now. I don't want folks to shake their heads at me or at Mama, pitying us for what we've sacrificed. That's like wet clothes I can't wait to take off because they're wrinkling my skin underneath. I just want to live my life.

I guess that's the best thing Judy Jones is teaching me. Just tell the stories. That's what she says to me. "You're sharing your story, Ms. Henry. That's the best thing you can do, for yourself and your loved ones," she says. "Keep it up."

I'm trying.

I'm taking Gunny out more too. We go hiking near what used to be Paradise Creek. He cracks me up because he won't stay on the trail with me. He goes the whole way splashing down the middle of the creek. When we get back home, his pads are waterlogged and he limps because they're puffy and tender. They wouldn't hurt him like that if he wouldn't soak them the whole way. It's okay, though, because he just plops down next to me for the rest of the day while I take my online class. I type and click and he licks his paws.

When I talked to Mama about her still praying for me it must have opened something up in her. She's been telling me more of what she's thinking. I'm not sure if that's good or not. Like the time she was doing dishes and she put down the mug in her hand and laid her towel over it. She walked close to me and said, "You're here, Kayla. That's what I want you to know. It's what I want, too. It's good that you're home. I want you to know that. I want you to act like you know that you are here. Home. Aren't you glad you're home?"

"No," I said. Just like that.

Her face crumpled. She asked, "How could you say that?"

I think it made me wake up a little. I said, "I'm sorry, Mama. Of course I'm glad I'm home." I followed her to the sink. I talked to her back.

"I know all this is supposed to mean 'home' to me, but it doesn't. My life in the Marines was straight-edged and clear. Which is weird, because, when I was in the middle of all that, deployed, all I wanted was to be here. But now that I am here, and everything around me is pine trees and rides to the post office, I don't know what to feel. Maybe you're right, Mama. Maybe I don't really feel like I'm here."

I don't think that explanation helped Mama. She was pretty quiet the rest of the night.

Pretty soon after our first appointments I figured out that Judy Jones was a strange therapist, or, at the very least, she had strange methods. But soon enough I also realized that she helped me anyway. Maybe she helped me because of her strangeness, so I kept seeing her. That, and she'd find me wherever I was and make me come to her office.

It was like her kookiness gave me permission to have my own quirks, too. That was refreshing after the military where I had to be just so and I couldn't even take a trip if I wanted. Now, if I want to just drop everything and go to Albuquerque or Phoenix, I do.

At first, Judy Jones warned me that my disappearing acts could be dangerous. Then she relaxed. She realized I wasn't going to do like my Dad and leave for good. She started giving me assignments for my trips: go to the science museum or check out a side street she recommended. She sent me to a weird neighborhood with nothing but Vietnamese cooking supply stores to eat weedy soup with sprouts. I loved every minute of it.

Once I stepped outside a bar where people sang barely adequate karaoke and these guys were kicking a little bald puppy, all spine and legs and nothing more. I lost it. I started picking up guys and throwing them on other ones, knocking them down like bowling pins. I'm probably lucky I didn't break anybody's back.

That's how I wound up with Grunt. He was the spindly puppy. My Iraq buddies think I named him after our nicknames as beginners in the military. That's not it. The poor guy was so tiny when I first picked him up. All he did was grunt like a piglet. How could I call him anything else?

Judy Jones says it wasn't good for me to almost break a bunch of puppy-kickers, even if they were nothing more than puppy-kickers. She says it's good for me to be sweet to little Grunt, though. I know she thinks it's good for both me and Grunt.

Gunny likes the pup. If he didn't, Gunny could put some mad hurt on Grunt pretty quick. Instead, I find Gunny and Grunt curled up together in Gunny's kennel. That won't work so well if Grunt gets much bigger.

I guess the day Judy Jones helped me the most was the day she kept pushing me to sum up my story of Iraq. I didn't know what she meant. How does anybody sum up their story of anything? You're too busy living it.

"Just tell your story," she kept at me. "Just tell it in fifty words or less!" Her voice got screechy and loud and she wouldn't stop.

"You can do it, if you really want to," Judy Jones said.

"What is there to say?" I finally asked. "My story is either a girl goes to war and comes back, or my story is a girl finds a boy, but he leaves her, just the way her dad did. Either way, so what?"

"The 'so what' is," she said. There was Therapist Voice again. ". . . Either way, it hurt you. That's enough."

We sat for another of the quiet spells between us. This time, Judy Jones didn't sit in a way that said she'd wait as long as it took. Her shoulders were up by her ears and she was leaning toward me with her elbows on her knees.

She said, "You mentioned that you used to be a chatterbox. Why aren't you anymore?"

"I grew up. Now I understand what people mean when they say some things are better left unsaid."

Judy Jones got past Therapist Voice and just talked to me normal. I'm learning that it's what comes after Therapist Voice that really teaches me something.

"Like any other saying, sure, that's true enough . . ." Judy Jones said, ". . . but it's dangerous if you take it too far. Some things, if you leave them unsaid, will kill you. It's not like talking to me or anybody else is a magic bullet, Ms. Henry. It's just that it's the only thing we've really got. It's like the saying about democracy, that it's the worst form of government except all the others. Talking's the worst way for us to fix ourselves, except for everything else we could try."

Then she, no kidding, stuck her tongue out and made a splat sound with her lips and she seemed to pause to see what I would do. What else could I do, I laughed like hell.

So, no, Judy Jones hasn't fixed me, but this week, before I went in to my appointment, I met Mama in the hallway. "Mama, I love you," I said. I hugged her and told her, "I'm glad to be home."

And I still haven't talked to Judy Jones, or Mama for that matter, about just what happened between me and Joe, but I'm getting closer.

PART IV

Relatives, Lovers, and Friends

The moral and in some cases legal obligation for parents to take care of children and children to take care of aging parents is the basis of much public policy and medical practice. There are of course exceptions when, either because of inability or unwillingness, these caregiving relationships are unfulfilled. The obligations of other people, related by blood or commitment, are not so clear. Yet they make up a substantial part of the caregiving population.

The stories in this section illustrate this aspect of family caregiving. Allegra Goodman's story "The Closet" is the story of two Chinese-American sisters in Hawaii. Lily, the child prodigy now an adult, refuses to come out of the closet at the top of the stairs. Evelyn, her sister, leaves meals for her and tries to coax her to come downstairs. In this story Evelyn's husband, who came from a "tall, meat-eating family in Providence, Rhode Island," is exasperated by both sisters' failure to address the problem forthrightly.

Two stories and one poem deal with the impact of the HIV/AIDS epidemic on families and friends. In Eugenia Collier's story "The Caregiver," the narrator is Donald's cousin. Donald has come home to take care of his demanding mother, Aunt Lou. The other members of Aunt Lou's family not only do not help out, they make their own demands on Donald, who is keeping secret his own illness because he fears that his African-American family and community will shun him.

"Oceanic Hotel, Nice," by Tereze Glück, is a story of the early years of the HIV/AIDS epidemic. The narrator tries to help Nicholas by visiting him in the hospital, sneaking him cigarettes, and cleaning his apartment. The narrator's dedication to caregiving wanes in the face of advancing illness. The obscure title becomes clear only at the very end of the story.

Mark Doty's poem "Atlantis" is a sequence of six poems about the illness of his lover Wally, who has AIDS ("not even a real word / but an acronym, a vacant / four-letter cipher") and the many friends affected by the epidemic. Their dog is a major character. "We don't have a future, / we have a dog." Wally too has dreams of "a light at the end" but then sees it as a reprieve. Their friend Michael, also a caregiver, dreams about helping Randy out of bed, becoming "a shining body, brilliant light / held in the form I first knew him in." Doty's chronicle of lost friends, and the lovers of lost friends, epitomizes the heartbreak of the epidemic as it unfolded on the East Coast.

28

The Closet

❧ *Allegra Goodman*

When she got home from work, Evelyn realized that her sister was now living full time in the closet. It was a big closet that spread out under the eaves. The house was built in the old Hawaiian style, two stories and white, with a long porch in front, and thick glass windows instead of louvres. There was even a cellar faced with stone—a rarity. Evelyn and her sister had a real old-fashioned Mainland house dug into the ground. In the thirties there had been a terraced garden. What remained was a macadamia-nut tree that pressed against the second-story windows. All the plants pressed on the house, damp leaves against the glass. The Manoa rains bent and warped the wooden doors. That morning, Evelyn had thought maybe her sister was stuck, that the closet door had jammed up there.

"Hit the top and pull the knob down at the same time," she called through the door. "Turn the knob and pull it down and hit the top above your head."

There was no answer.

That afternoon, when Evelyn walked in from the bus stop, the house was still. Lily's clothes and her books had been neatly cleared out of the rest of the house. Her toothbrush and even her old piano music were gone. The music rack and the piano bench were empty.

Lily had often gone up to the closet during the day. They were used to that. Lily was ill. Her illness had many shifting names and ambiguities. Her actions, however, seemed to become more pointed and specific every year. She would not drive. Then she would not leave the house. She would not cook or play the piano, pick up the telephone, or answer the door. Now, it seemed, she would not come downstairs.

Evelyn told her husband about it when he came home. "Should we call the doctor?" she asked him. "Should we call Roselva?" Roselva was Lily's caseworker from the Hawaii Department of Human Services.

"Oh, for God's sake," Stan said.

"I'm sorry," Evelyn said, and she was sorry. It was hard on Stan, living with his sister-in-law in such a state.

"She's forty-nine years old," Stan said, and he paced around the living room.

Evelyn looked at him nervously. She was afraid Stan would blow his top. Lily had always been afraid of him. Stan came from a tall, meat-eating family in Providence, Rhode Island. He grew up wearing shoes in a dark house on a hill, a house rattling with storms and icicles. Evelyn personally had never seen it in winter, but the picture was there in her mind, the ice and snowdrifts.

Evelyn made spring rolls with fresh mint leaves for dinner. She steamed some rice and made mock duck and spicy vegetarian meatballs, which her sister loved. She set the table and opened the double doors between the living room and the dining room. Soon the scent would fill the house; it would drift up the stairs into every corner. She imagined somehow that the scent would drift up from her to Lily. It would be like the incense in their Chinese uncle's little temple in Kaimuki. She and Lily used to go there when they were children. They would smell the incense sticks and the candles in the shrine by the brown runoff canal trailing down to the ocean. Now a light haze of smoke drifted from the cooling wok in the kitchen.

Evelyn went to get Stan, and she found him in the basement. He was cracking a macadamia nut in the vise. It was the only way; they were so hard. "Dinner," she said.

They ate by themselves. Afterward, Evelyn took up spring rolls, mock duck, meatballs, rice, and a pitcher of iced tea on a tray for Lily. She left the tray by the closet door. The food was gone in the morning. Only a few rice grains were left.

She started leaving food out every night. Saimin on the hot plate, tofu-and-alfalfa sandwiches on sprouted-wheat rolls, vegetarian Manapua from work. Evelyn worked in Ala Moana Shopping Center at the Golden Apple—famous for selling vegetarian whole food. Evelyn had created a lot of the Golden Apple's recipes. She had been in the vegetarian-shiatsu-acupuncture community for years and had pioneered several techniques for taking the meat, fat, and cholesterol out of Hawaiian food. Admittedly, the vegetarian version often bore no resemblance to the original. Real Manapua—the kind kids bought after school—were big white dumplings, soft and glutinous, made of flour and lard, with a little pork in the center and a red mark on the round surface like the chop mark of a brush painter. Evelyn's whole-wheat-and-bean dumplings were nothing like this. Still, they had their following at the takeout counter. She brought extras home for her sister. She put out her homemade almond cookies and cold drinks.

Each morning the food was gone. Lily didn't speak to her from inside the closet. She made no sign that she intended to move back into her own room.

When Lily had been living up in the closet for a week, Stan got nervous, because he needed to get an estimate from the exterminators. He had already scheduled the appointment. The termite control team had to look at the whole house—and especially the closet. They had to get in there and assess the damage.

"Maybe it can wait," Evelyn suggested as they ate breakfast.

"It's waited thirty years," Stan said. "It's waiting that caused all this in the first place! We've got dry rot, mold, silverfish, beetles. They're talking about a tent job."

"If it's waited thirty years, it can wait a little longer," Evelyn said.

"We've got some walls in the bathroom, they're only paint," Stan said, and he stared over Evelyn's head at the damp rotting part of the wall where he envisioned a gaping hole above the utility sink. He looked down at the worn wooden floor, which was damp and, he thought, chewed up.

"Don't be upset," Evelyn said.

She didn't know what else to say. Stan hadn't wanted to move into the old house in the first place. Evelyn thought maybe the Mainland-style basement brought back unhappy memories for him. Maybe it reminded him of his father, whom he grew up disappointing. His father was a famous theoretical physicist, a big professor at Brown. He studied the structure of the universe and expected his only son to do the same. Stan was no good at it, and ran away to join the Air Force so he could be a pilot. He was going to fly fighter planes, screaming off into the sky from aircraft carriers, but in the end the Air Force decided to send him to Hawaii to be a meteorologist.

"Your parents just let this place rot away." Stan got up from the table.

As Evelyn washed the breakfast dishes, she looked out the window over the sink to where their fence had been. In a storm last winter the fence, hollowed out by termites, had floated up light as a glider and fallen softly into paint splinters in the neighbor's bougainvillea. But what did a fence matter? It was a good house. It was roomy. It had wood floors. How could it be rotten inside? Evelyn couldn't believe Stan when he said that. The place had ceilings high above even Stan's head.

Evelyn and Lily had come to their grandparents' house with some awe as children. It seemed ancient to them. The koa-wood floors were cool and smooth against their bare feet. Everything cool that way was old. Then, years later, when Evelyn and Lily inherited the place, Lily said she was glad Stan and Evelyn were going to live there with her. She said she would be afraid to live there alone. Five years ago, Evelyn and Stan had unpacked and taken the master bedroom. They had never owned even half a house before. They'd raised their daughter, Anna, in an apartment near the Ala Wai canal. The balcony there was only big enough for two chairs and Anna's bicycle. The kitchen appliances in that apartment were the color people called avocado. It was really more the color of guacamole left in the refrigerator, or the tint of canned asparagus.

Evelyn began to come home from work earlier, gradually, almost imperceptibly—a few minutes earlier each day. With a pounding heart she turned her key in the lock. As softly as she could, she pushed open the swollen front door. There was always a cracking sound as the door swung open, no matter what she did. But she slipped off her sandals and hurried in, half expecting to see Lily on the stairs or catch sight of her in the kitchen. She listened for footsteps; her eyes darted over the living room. She hoped to see her sister downstairs, but the hope was mixed up now with a kind of fear because she hadn't seen her for so long.

She imagined Lily cutting open the papayas Stan kept on the counter. Or watching television five hours at a time, curled up in the leaky bean-bag chair that was Anna's before she went to college. Walking through the house in her little tabbies. Lily was small, like Evelyn. They both had size-5 feet. She even imagined Lily instructing yoga classes in the living room. That had been her profession years ago. She would bend, and breathe, and walk around the room, watching her students. Tense shoulders would dissolve at her touch. Clenched muscles would melt. She imagined Lily sitting down at the piano, a lovely Yamaha ruined by the humidity, and playing Chopin in her own curious way, as if she had serious reservations about where the music was going. Lily had soloed with the Honolulu Symphony in 1950, when she was nine, a great event for the family. Evelyn watched as Lily received a three-strand ilima lei from Tutu and a money lei from Auntie Maude, dollar bills folded into flowers and strung into a beautiful green mass. Evelyn got a crisp two-strand pikake lei that hung like a long pearl necklace. After an hour the lei was limp on her neck. It smelled so sweet the fragrance seemed to wring out and exhaust the flowers. She got that lei after Lily's performance, because she was the sister.

But where was Lily now? Maybe in the mornings she snuck out of the house altogether, slipped down the street and took the bus. She could get all the way around the island if she transferred in Waikiki. All the way around, or almost, for seventy-five cents. They used to take the two-hour trip in rattling buses from the Y.M.C.A. summer camp. Every summer they went on that field trip. Lily and Evelyn were on different buses, of course, with their age groups. In swimming class Evelyn was a Polliwog, while Lily had already passed her Fish test. Evelyn was waiting to become a Fish. She was waiting to get to the blue piano book and the green reading level, and backflips.

Evelyn began to make mistakes at work. She nearly scalded herself with hot oil at the deep fryers. She cut her finger slicing sweet potato and forgot the extra crackle batter for the tempura. She got behind on the orders, because all the time she was wondering, Was Lily eating pistachios on the living room floor? Shelling them into the wastebasket? Was she taking a long bath—washing her hair, leaning back in the tub?

"What's wrong wit' you?" her boss asked her. He was a young kid just graduated from U.H.

"My sister's moved into the closet." Evelyn sighed.

"The closet? How come?"

"I don't know," Evelyn said.

"Whoa," her boss said. "She came out of the closet, and then she went back in?"

On her way to the bus stop each morning, Evelyn began walking back to the house, as if she'd forgotten something. Then she started rushing home in the middle of the day. She thought somehow she could get home when Lily wouldn't expect it. She would meet her on the stairs; she would sit down next to her at the kitchen table, and they would talk. It had to happen, sooner or later. Evelyn left work early; she came late. Every day, she tried her luck, testing the odds like a gambler. In the end, she lost her job.

The day her boss fired her, Evelyn stood in her mother's kitchen and brewed a pot of green popcorn tea. This was a strange but soothing drink; green tea with tiny bits of popcorn floating in it. The tea came from a Chinese store in Kaimuki, where they often had dinner at the King's Garden. They would walk home in the warm twilight past Harry's Music Store, where Lily's music came from—the hardest kind, in manila covers and with black printing, whole chains of tiny black notes, whole archipelagoes.

"I never liked that job," Evelyn explained to Stan when he got home. "I've been thinking about it for a long time. I want to go back and finish my degree. I've just got one more year, and there's a real shortage of chiropractors right now; there's a real need."

"I've got a real need for your sister to get out of that closet," Stan said.

Evelyn gave Stan a back rub. She laid him down on the living-room floor and rolled him out on his back and massaged his ankles. She poked the soles of his feet with the eraser end of a pencil. She knew Stan was thinking about money. She knew he was worrying about the termites. The exterminators were on hold until Lily came down. And no one but Lily knew when that would be. It wasn't a question of asking Lily or reasoning with her. It was one of those things you couldn't change. Like fate. Like the weather. Of course, Stan knew all about the weather; he was a meteorologist. But he hadn't wanted to be one.

At night, in bed, Evelyn could almost hear the bugs chewing the house away. She could hear the soft thuds of the cockroaches flying in the kitchen, batting against the walls. Mold and damp crept over the bathroom tiles. She and Lily had inherited a house dissolving like a white sugar cube into the tropical soil, a succulent white house. Long ago, the termites had begun colonizing the cabinets; the ants wove in and out, exploring. For years, ferns had been growing on the garage roof. A lush canopy of ferns and deep-green moss. The house had a life of its own. Tenting the whole place would be a custom job. The tent would be rolled out and clipped right onto the house, over the roof, around all the corners. The house would have to be wrapped up like a Christmas present for the fumigators, sealed up so none of the bugs and poison would escape. It would cost four thousand dollars, plus their hotel bills while the house was sealed away. They didn't have that kind of money. It wasn't just Lily holding them up.

She lay in bed and imagined Lily curled up in the dark closet like the curled-up frond of a tree fern furled into its tight, secret knot. She imagined Lily gliding up and down the stairs, opening the cupboards, her hair swinging behind her, batting softly against the walls.

The kids came home for winter break and ran through the house like giants. The kids were Anna, their daughter, and her boyfriend, Mike. They were both music-education majors at the University of Puget Sound, and they sang together and banged on the piano. Clouds of dust rose wherever they walked.

Anna sat in the kitchen and caught the flying cockroaches in her bare hands and threw them out the door. Anna was big, like Stan. Almost six feet. She had hazel eyes, and hair so thick and long it stood out like a brown cloud around her shoulders. When she braided it down, it bounced back up. She'd inherited the hair from the Hawaiian side of Evelyn's family.

With the kids around, Stan moved differently. His shoulders weren't tight, and he didn't tense up in his neck. Anna was his baby. He'd set out to raise her without the pressure he'd had as a child. Stan had always told Anna—ever since she was three years old—"Listen, no one's telling you what to do, where to go, what kind of person to be." Anna didn't understand all this when she was three, but she did grow up extremely calm. They had raised her without a bedtime and without a curfew, and she was, tall and mellow, as some girls are when they grow up with lots of boyfriends and few rules. Anna and Mike spent their days out at the beach. Fine sand spread over the kitchen floorboards and in between the cushions of the couch.

When Evelyn left dinner for Lily by the closet door, Anna came upstairs with her. "Hi, Auntie," she called through the door, "Come out soon. We miss you. The piano is lonely."

"Anna," Stan said at dinner. "It's no joke. Auntie has got Mom waiting on her hand and foot."

"I guess she likes it in there," Anna said. At her side, Mike ate steadily.

Evelyn dreamed that night that she was inside the closet. She'd forgotten how big it was. There was an antique sofa and a phonograph, a pair of tap shoes, and a stack of books up to the round porthole window. "Little Women" and "Doctor Doolittle," twelve Oz books and algebra texts. Lily sat in a wicker rocking chair in there, crocheting.

A scream woke Evelyn. It took her breath away. Lily! she thought. Stan sprang up. They rushed downstairs and nearly collided with Lily, wide-eyed in the pale light of the open refrigerator. Mike stood naked at the kitchen door.

Mike looked around bewildered, sunburned and hairy. "I was hungry," he said.

"Lily!" Evelyn said. "Please. I want to talk to you." But Lily had already started to run.

"Lily! Lily!" Stan yelled, and he scrambled after her up the stairs. He caught at her wrist, but she pulled away so hard he lost his balance and fell. Lily rushed up the stairs and out of sight.

"Stan, you scared her!" Evelyn said. She looked at Stan and Mike. "You scared her. Both of you."

Mike was still standing there naked. What was wrong with him? Why didn't he put something on? Where was Anna?

Anna had slept through the whole thing.

Stan took off from work and made phone calls. He stayed home the next day, too, so that he and Evelyn could talk with Roselva, the social worker.

Roselva came and embraced them both. She wore a red muumuu, and carried Lily's files in a canvas Honolulu Academy of Arts tote bag.

They sat down together in the living room.

"Do you think she's in danger?" Roselva asked.

"In danger? Of course not," Stan said. "She's not exactly starving. She comes down, we think, to use the facilities. But not when we're around."

Roselva took some notes. "Do you think she's afraid of something?"

"No," Evelyn said.

"Well, I'll go and try to talk to her," said Roselva. Stan got up, but she shook her head. "I think she'll want to speak to me privately," she said, and she walked up the stairs.

Stan and Evelyn sat in the living room and strained their ears. They heard the creak of the stairs and the squeak of the second-floor landing. "You think she's really going to come out and talk to her?" Evelyn asked Stan.

"Not a chance," Stan said.

But half an hour passed. Evelyn stood by the front window and watched the light rain drift in a mist down the street. Birds splashed in pools of water between the roots of the macadamia-nut tree. In the winter she and Lily used to go mudsliding near Paradise Park, up at Jackass Ginger. They took torn cardboard boxes and hiked up, ankle deep in mud. They grasped the slick stems of the giant philodendrons, they ducked under the twisting vines. Invisible birds flew overhead among the leaves. There was a trickle of water, a hum of mosquitoes. When they got to the top they flung themselves down on the flattened boxes. Covered with mud, they trudged back up again, scratched their mosquito bites, slicked their hair back in muddy waves. Hidden beyond the trees was the cool pure reservoir, deep, clear, and forbidden.

"Well," Roselva said. She startled Evelyn and Stan as she came back into the living room.

"She came out?" Stan asked.

"She came out," said Roselva.

"What did she say?" Evelyn asked. "What does she want?"

"She wants to stay where she is." Roselva shut her notebook. "I know this is very hard for you."

"Isn't there something you can do?" Stan asked.

"Well," Roselva said. "The state can't just go up there and police her life style."

"Life style! But she's sick," Stan said.

"Yes, she is ill, but she does have rights," Roselva said.

"So my wife has to spend her nights cooking for this woman? This is a manipulative recluse we have up there," Stan said. "This is a woman with a bunker mentality. What if she goes berserk one night? What if she decides to burn the house down?"

"There are groups—for families," Roselva said. "There are resources. I know this is a big adjustment to make."

"We can't adjust to this," Stan said. "We can't live like this."

"But the fact is," Roselva said, "she's in no danger, either to herself or to the family. There is no sign of drug abuse, sexual abuse, or alcoholism. She's not a runaway, of course."

"No!" Stan threw up his hands. "It's just the opposite!" And of course this was true. Lily was not a runaway. Somehow she had done the other thing. Somehow she had gone into internal exile. At the top of the house she had become a stowaway.

Rain washed the valley green. It ran down green ridges into tiny waterfalls and rivulets and then into Manoa Stream. The ground was soft, the black streets sparkled. Anna and Mike came home that night pink with the sun from the beach in Waimanalo. "You guys should come with us tomorrow," Mike said.

"It's not raining out there," Anna told them.

"We'll see," Stan said. He glanced up at the ceiling in his aggravation, as if Lily could see them. But the next day was Saturday, so they went.

Early in the morning, Evelyn packed a cooler with tofu sandwiches, carrot and celery sticks, grapes, bottled water, tangerines, and Maui potato chips. She took a bottle of meat tenderizer as well—to rub on in case someone was stung by jellyfish. Then, at the last minute, she ran up the stairs to the closet door. "Lily, do you want to come to the beach?" she asked. "I think it would be good for you to get out of the house. Get some exercise."

She waited, but there was no response. "I'm leaving you some fruit," she said. She left a little pyramid of tangerines by the door.

They drove out to the other side of the island, and the sea spread out green before them, violet-blue in the distance. The sky was dry and distant, as if rain had never existed.

When they unfurled their tatami mats, the white sand whipped up and sent tiny, almost transparent crabs scurrying into new holes. Anna and Mike plunged into the surf, bobbing and paddling out into the waves. The wet sand sucked up their leaping footprints. Evelyn followed them slowly. She stood where the waves broke at her waist. The air was sweet and salty, like dried salted plums. Maybe they should stop and buy some on the way home. They always used to stop on the way home from the beach and finger the racks of dried seeds. There was dried lemon peel; you peeled it open and picked out the bitter seeds before you ate it, tangy and salt-dusted. There were bags of shredded ginger, wet and fibrous mango strips, juicy black rocksalt plums you sucked until the pits scraped your palate, dried kumquats, plump and tart. I should get some for Lily, she thought as she bobbed over the waves.

On shore, Stan slept, out among the sea grapes, eyes shut, zinc oxide on his nose. The kids were swimming away, paddling farther out like a pair of Irish setters. And, in between, Evelyn stood in the water. She was still thinking about Lily. She couldn't help it, even out there in the ocean. Lily lived now in her mind, with her piano and her yoga mats and her lunchbox from school, her books, her tap shoes—she'd set up housekeeping. When Evelyn swam, Lily was swimming. When she dreamed, Lily was dreaming. Always, her sister was with her. The memory of her filled Evelyn. Every tiny eyelash of her. The touch of her dog-eared piano music, paper worn soft as cloth, the origami boxes that she had made, the school uniforms, Black Watch plaid and white short-sleeved shirts and sandals. The firecrackers on New Year's at the splintering old temple with its litchi tree, the ground carpeted with red wrappers and litchis. They were all there inside Evelyn. They filled her to the brim, the tiniest details of her sister. No matter how she tried, she could not stop thinking about Lily. It was because she would never get her back.

No one but Evelyn knew anymore what Lily used to be. No one else knew the record and the history of her brilliant life—all her accomplishments, playing the piano and swimming, all her days. They lasted only in Evelyn's memory. No one else could picture them. That was the worst thing for Evelyn—that somehow she was the last of her sister's family and friends, the last of the listeners from those old recitals, and the Young People's Concert with the Symphony, when Lily played in her muumuu with her tiny perfect fingers, her hair braided in two glossy braids. Her sound was big and serene. She was like a jockey riding that black concert-grand piano. Now all the applause was gone, and all that hope; and that old Lily, the one Evelyn so looked up to, now lived in Evelyn's head.

Evelyn stood waist deep in the ocean, and she jumped over the crests of the incoming waves. She kicked her feet at the smooth sand under her. "Get out of my head," she called into the wind. And she thought, Stay in the closet but get out of my head. She didn't mind bringing dinner to the closet door, or taking away the dirty plates; she didn't mind, even if Lily came downstairs while they were asleep. None of that mattered. It was the old thoughts and feelings that welled up inside her. The memories that rose up. That was what was hard to bear. She watched the kids bobbing in the distance. She took a deep breath and let it out slowly. She breathed out, as if she could blow Lily back into the world. Lily believed in breathing. It was the center of yoga. Breathing was the most important thing.

Shivering, Evelyn walked in onto the beach, and the white foam licked her heels. The ocean rose up behind her. Big, but not big enough.

Tight-wrapped lumpia boiled up to the top of the bubbling oil, and Evelyn skimmed them out with her open wire ladle. The kids were already sitting at the table. Evelyn set aside four lumpia on a paper towel for Lily and took them upstairs with a little dish of sauce. "It's ridiculous," Stan was telling the kids downstairs. "Ridiculous." Evelyn knelt down and put the plate of lumpia by the door. She didn't feel ridiculous. That wasn't the word. She was exhausted and trembling, hot with sunburn between her shoulders. She was aching. But they ate dinner as usual, watched the news on television. The kids went out to a movie. Stan said the sun had done him good.

At night, when she was falling asleep, Evelyn felt the rise and fall of the waves against her body. It had always been that way when they spent the day at the beach. The rhythm of the waves stayed with her, washed over her. She dreamed she was jumping waves with Lily. She dreamed of the nights after those long jumps over waves. How she and Lily would fall asleep with the waves still rushing against them. And the waves rose up in their beds, and the two of them kept on leaping, kicking up the sand, and springing over the white water, heads up over the tangled crests of the waves.

Evelyn woke for a moment and then felt herself falling asleep again. She knew the dream would still be there.

29

The Caregiver

 Eugenia Collier

O God, O God, if she doesn't stop that damn racket I'm going to beat her uncon-scious! No, no, no! My mother . . . Mother . . . old, sick. Something wrong with me, thinking like that. SHUT UP, LOU, HUSH HOLLERING! I'll come in there and make you hush, dammit—

In the background I could hear Aunt Lou shrieking at Donald. "I don't know what I'm going to do with her," Donald was saying above the confu-sion. "She won't even let me talk on the phone anymore. If I leave her room she starts hollering like that and keeps on until I hang up and come back in there with her."

"She sounds pretty strong to me," I said. How could anyone so sick make all that noise?

"What? I can't hear you."

"Look, Donald, I don't know what to tell you," I yelled into the phone. "You can't go on living like this. She's going to . . . ."

"Sister Little, I can't talk now," he said, reverting to the name they used to call me when we were children. Even though I wasn't anybody's sister but Manny's, and slightly taller, though he was older, the family used to call me Sister Little. "I'll get back to you after she goes to sleep."

I went back to the lecture I was preparing for my next day's Ameri-can Lit class, and when, sometime later, I looked at the clock, it was well past eleven. He hadn't called. Figuring that he had probably fallen asleep when Aunt Lou did, I didn't call him. What could I say to him anyway? He wasn't going to put his mother into a nursing home, and they couldn't afford full-time care—or even much part-time care—in their house. Don-ald had taken early retirement from his job in New York, and his pension and Aunt Lou's together didn't go far. So Donald was nurse, housekeeper, cook, and companion. He fed her, bathed her, changed her diapers, and listened to her wild ramblings.

What could I say to him? There was only one possible solution, and we both knew it. My problem and that of my brother Manny was solved that way five years ago: Our mother had died.

Sleep—finally. Looks so little lying there. Lemme tuck the cover around her shoulders. So thin. There. Lord, I'm tired! Got to wash the dishes before I go to bed. What am I gonna do, what, what? Hope I can sleep tonight. What am I gonna do? Thought just goes round and round in my brain like one of those crazy rides in a carnival. God!

Two or three weeks passed before I called Donald again. Knowing that his tight budget wouldn't permit many long-distance calls, even between Washington and Baltimore, I usually called him. Aunt Lou was quiet this time.

"She had a good day," Donald reported. "Ate a good dinner. But she always eats pretty good." He sighed.

"And how are you doing?" I asked. He had been ailing lately. I suspected, though, that Donald had more than a touch of hypochondria, a malady from which a number of our relatives suffered.

"Not the best. My stomach stays upset, and I keep having pains in my back."

"Maybe it's your nerves."

"Maybe. I'm going to the doctor Friday if I can find somebody to sit with Lou."

We talked for a while about how, with so much family nearby, there was never anybody to come and spend a few hours with Lou so that he could attend to other matters. Whenever he could get away, our Aunt Etta, who lived alone, would prevail upon him to do her supermarket shopping. Etta had a grown son, but she hadn't brought him up, having lost custody in a particularly bitter divorce when he was a little boy, and he lived somewhere in California. Etta had grown old alone. She shared with her brothers and sisters the conviction that family members were obliged to meet each other's needs, totally and without question. For her the obligation went one way: She demanded much and gave nothing. Like her brother Horace, she was frequently hospitalized for depression. After one such confinement, not wanting to be alone, she went to spend a few days with Horace and his wife Gladys. She stayed for ten years, until Gladys issued the ultimatum, "Either she goes, or I do."

"Ask Etta to stay with Aunt Lou," I suggested wickedly.

"Yeah—when pigs fly and jaybirds swim." It was an old expression that we had used years ago when we were kids at Grandma's. Suddenly I saw him as he had been then—hazel eyes and crinkly sandy hair, skin golden in the sunshine, face lit up with mischief. The flash of memory both cheered and depressed me.

We talked for a few more minutes, then he asked, "How's Manny getting along?" as he always did, and I replied, "Fine," as I always did, and we hung up. But the image of the child Donald hovered in my mind like the phantom ache of an amputated limb.

From a TV camera long shot, our childhood would have appeared idyllic—three country kids playing merrily in a large fenced-in yard ringed by berry bushes and dotted with fruit trees. As the camera panned closer, however, it would have revealed small stresses not associated with childhood joy: the spastic gait of the smallest child, the hunched shoulders and spindly limbs of the girl. An extreme closeup would perhaps focus on our faces, and the viewer might read there the silent, separate tragedies that would mark our lives.

My brother Manny had cerebral palsy, the result of a birth injury. I was born a year later. The family believed that God had sent me to take care of my brother. The "normal" child, I was orphaned by my brother's need.

Our mother having suffered a "nervous breakdown" during our pre-school years, we spent long periods at her parents' home on the outskirts of Washington, D.C. At other times we lived with our father's parents in Baltimore, where daddy was a young physician building a practice. In a sense, we were nomads, belonging nowhere.

Donald was our cousin, our Aunt Lou's child. Ours was a large extended family—our mother was the oldest of nine—and uncles, aunts, and cousins were constantly in and out of the white frame house which was the family's hub. Donald was a frequent visitor, and the three of us, Donald, Manny, and I, were steady companions. Donald was like an older brother. His presence lightened the gloom that characterized our life in that place. We did childish things—gorged ourselves on Granddaddy's gooseberries, captured bees in jars, ran haphazardly over the lawn, told stories of fantastic adventures, built a "Fu Manchu" dummy out of a broom and our uncle's old clothes, of which we pretended to be terrified as Donald and I dashed past, screaming. Sometimes Donald drew pictures for us on scrap paper. Our mischief was mild, for we were "good" children, obedient and perhaps even intimidated by the adult world.

There was reason for our intimidation. Our family was descended from house slaves—although nobody ever admitted our slave past until a cousin seeking roots dug up the dirt. The copious white blood of which they were so proud had given them not only white skin and wavy hair but also a genetic form of depression. Ours was a nervous, quarrelsome family—handsome, intelligent, relatively affluent, but tainted with neurosis. Terribly ingrown, the members of our family had few friends outside of each other, and their relationships with each other were often destructive. It was a family of controlling women and passive men. The women consumed their sons and alienated their daughters. It wasn't that they didn't love us. It was only that love was encased in a kernel of warped emotions. The result was a family afflicted with astigmatism of the mind's eye, which perceived a world of distorted images. This was the world of our childhood.

I never knew Donald's father. Aunt Lou married in her teens and had her only child at seventeen. Charley Hope soon faded out of the family. An aunt once told me that Lou considered herself less attractive than her sisters, lacking their "good" hair and Caucasian features, and had married out of defiance. In any case, Aunt Lou reared her son alone, and in the old family tradition, possessed him fiercely. She never remarried, and if she ever had a steady boyfriend, I never knew. Donald called his mother by her first name—she wasn't much older than he.

Donald continued to be our close companion throughout our early years. For me he filled a special need: an older brother who was not engulfed in my mother's obsession, my father's frustration, and my own ambivalence. In our family we never talked about Manny's cerebral palsy. Neither he nor I understood his condition; nobody had ever explained it to us. I knew only that our parents' emotional resources were focused on him. My role was to serve. So, I think now, I needed the brother I found in Donald.

And perhaps Donald needed siblings as much as I needed him. Perhaps the children of dysfunctional families have a way of banding together in unconscious alliance against a hurtful world. In any case, his presence made me happy. His quick imagination, his keen humor, and his gentleness made his visits occasions for celebration. Manny and I started school in Washington, where our mother taught in an elementary school. Still living at Grandma's house during the week, we saw Donald frequently. After we transferred to a Baltimore school in the fourth grade, our parents having bought a house in Baltimore (although our mother still taught in Washington), we saw Donald less frequently, but his visits were high points in our lives. Gradually they became less frequent, and in the frenzy of the high school years, we lost touch.

I rerun memories like old movies. At night I come upstairs and fall across my bed and sleep like something dead; then all of a sudden I'm sitting up at some godless hour staring in the dark. I undress then and pour a little scotch and water and get under the covers and sip and close my eyes. I see Lou the way she used to be when I was a little boy. She used to fuss at me a lot—I can hear that screechy voice of hers giving me hell—but she took care of me. After Charley left, it was just her and me. Grandma and the aunts used to say, "You ought never forget your mother. She stuck by you. You ought never forget her." Sometimes I'd hear them talking to each other about my father. "Charley Hope is about as low-down a nigger as niggers come. Wasn't for his color and his good hair, he wouldn't have nothing." Charley. I remember him only in fragments, like a dream that dims in waking. But Lou, my mother, stuck by me.

By the second scotch I'm seeing all those years in New York. Lord, didn't Lou have a fit when I told her I'd gotten a job in New York! Seemed so far away then. Laid a real guilt trip on me, they did—Lou and Grandma and them. But after Lou'd broke up my thing with Edith, I knew I couldn't stay. Hell, I was up in my twenties then and she was still asking me where I was going when I went out. New York—good years. Negroes and white people all mixed up together, didn't matter which was which. Art school in the evenings—yes, then finally the job I really wanted. The apartment with Jerry and Alvin—images come sweet and fast.

By the third scotch I can think about Stuart. The first years, anyway. The memory-movie slows now, and I see those years in slow motion. I examine them for details I might have forgotten—colors, gestures, voice textures, a touch of hands—not in any order but just the way they come. Until the end when he is white as dough, shriveled, a skeleton covered with splotchy skin, a skeleton with red fire in the eye sockets, and he opens his flame-red mouth, and I hear Lou screaming, and I jolt awake, my face wet with tears.

Donald sold their house that spring and moved them into a sunny little house in Maryland, right outside Washington, closer to some of the relatives. One Sunday our Uncle Horace's wife Gladys met us at Donald's house, and the three of us went out to dinner. It was rare that Donald and Gladys were both available: She was usually afraid to leave Horace alone these days, but she had taken a chance today, and Donald had asked a friend to stay with Aunt Lou. Gladys was only a few years older than we were, and we enjoyed each other's company immensely.

After dinner Gladys hurried home, and Donald showed me around the new house. We talked awhile in his tiny room upstairs, where Aunt Lou had never been. I wondered at the neatness of the room, as if nobody spent any time there.

"Did you do these?" I asked, standing in the doorway, surveying the paintings that covered the walls.

"I did them when I was in New York. I painted a lot then."

There were several landscapes and a couple of seascapes. They were fairly straightforward realistic works, but there was grace in the sweep of wind in the grass, in the clouds over the mountains, in the waves lapping at the shore. One seascape especially held my gaze. A sailboat was battered by winds, and no shore was in sight. The sails were tattered. Furious waves swept the deck; the little boat listed badly, about to capsize. The colors were dark and ominous—purples, deep blues, blacks. The painting was a recapitulation of my own stormy moods.

The painting on the wall above his bed was more cheerful, and I turned to it with relief. It was a portrait of a young man grinning broadly, his maroon shirt and off-white scarf radiating joy. Despite his wavy dark hair and flashing eyes, the young man was not exactly handsome, but he looked like someone you would like to know. He must have been standing in the sun, for he was circled by a beam of light.

"Oh, I really like this one," I exclaimed. "Who is this? A friend of yours?"

Donald smiled briefly. "A friend of mine in New York. He's dead now."

"Oh." I wanted to ask more, but Donald's tone told me to leave it alone. I sat down on the edge of the bed, and he dropped wearily into a chair.

"I can't paint anymore," he said softly, leaning back, his eyes closed.

"No time?"

He shook his head slowly. "No peace."

"Oh Donald, isn't there something you can do with Aunt Lou?"

"What else is there to do? The woman from the agency comes for a couple of hours every other day. That's something. Actually, some days she doesn't show. I get to do the shopping—Etta's too—and that's about it."

"All those aunts who persuaded you to come back to Washington to take care of her—don't they ever help?"

"Huh! They're older than she is, except Etta, and she's never going to help anybody." Gingerly I approached a subject we had discussed before. "What about a nursing home?"

"Sister Little, I just can't do that."

"Why not?" But I knew why not. Every fiber of me knew it. I recalled the agony of luring my mother into my car and rushing her to a nursing home. I remembered the indignity of giving the admissions officer her bank book to copy; they knew exactly how long it would take to "spend down" until nothing was left. Nothing for Manny to live on. Nothing. I remembered my tears. She had been a very private person, and I knew that exposing her business to strangers would have caused her pain. I remembered the odor of old urine. I remembered the sight of my mother, a woman of great dignity, even in her dementia, tied to a chair because otherwise she wandered all over the home and once even escaped for three hellish hours. All of this, ever just below the surface of my thought, flashed across my mind in the instant between my question and his answer.

"Because I can't. I talked to Gladys and Horace about it. They don't believe in putting old folks in nursing homes. They took care of Grandma, and after she dies, they took care of Gladys's mother. They didn't put them into any nursing home."

"But they worked together, pooled their strength. Horace was a lot better then."

"Well, all the aunts say Lou is my responsibility. And they're right. You know how they carried on when you put your mother away."

"I didn't put her away. She needed care. Manny couldn't take care of her. She was doing some really bizarre things, and he certainly couldn't run after her when she got out of the house. He was in a wheelchair by then. You know that."

"They said you'd abandoned your mother."

That hurt. My mother had always expected me to live with them so that I could take care of my brother when she was too old. It had been a tremendous struggle for me to marry and move out, and after the marriage ended, to continue to live on my own. "I didn't abandon her," I told Donald angrily. "I had a full-time job, a house, and a life. What was I supposed to do? Give up my whole life to be a twenty-four-hour, seven-day nurse?"

"That's what I did."

I didn't say, "Yeah, and look what it got you." We were both in too much pain. Neither of us was much good at quarreling. We eased down to a safer subject—something fairly trivial—and I started back to Baltimore, depressed.

I'd just as well have died when I came back to Washington. My life, over anyway. Stuart—gone. All my time, taking her back and forth to one doctor or another. Never got better, only worse. Cranky and mean—nothing I did for her ever enough. No such thing as a thank you. Had to know where I was going, who with, and for how long—even if I wasn't going anywhere but to the store. Damn, I had turned sixty, and my mother still hassling me. "Donald, do this. . . . Donald, do that. . . . Hand me this. . . . Get me that." I liketa went crazy, too. Got worse. Started doing her business everywhere. I had to clean up shit. Had to bathe her, wash my mother's pussy. Who else was there to do it but

me? If anybody did come see about her—the aunts or uncles or anybody—nobody ever said she was clean and the house didn't stink. Nobody ever said, "Donald, you're doing a good job, can I help?" Nobody really looked at me. The lesions that were beginning to come on my hands and face—nobody even noticed. O God, my back!

❧

I don't know when or how I first realized that Donald was gay. Back when we were in our teens I heard some of the aunts call him a sissy behind his back. In our family we never talked about things like that. We never talked about sex anyway. Sex was dirty and only low-class niggers did it. Or, at least, only low-class niggers enjoyed it.

It didn't matter to me whether or not Donald was gay. We were cousins, we had shared a childhood, and even though we seldom saw each other, he was stability in my life. During those lonely growing-up years I had never felt loved—or even worthy of love—in the adult world. My value was my ability to serve. What we shared—Donald, Manny, and I—was like a full moon on a starless night. What did it matter whether Donald was gay?

We love where we can.

❧

If she would just die! Driving me crazy! Mornings when I go into her room—still alive! Still alive! STOP IT! STOP THAT HOLLERING! SHUT UP! SHUT UP! I'LL SHUT YOU UP! O my God! My fingers around her throat! Her eyes, looking at me like that! Dark holes. Her tongue, slimy, spit all over her face! O God! Upstairs, got to get out of here! Lou hollering and me beating my head against the wall and crying until her voice is gone and all my pain converges in my bloodied head.

❧

"What did the doctor say?" I asked Donald the next time he called.

"Says I've got a chronic liver infection."

"Damn. Are you taking antibiotics?"

"Yes, she gave me some medicine."

"Oh, Donald. All the stress. You're in your sixties. Somebody ought to be taking care of *you!*"

"The doctor gave me some tranquilizers. The headaches are better. I'm supposed to go back in two weeks if I can get somebody to stay with Lou."

I suppressed the thought that I hated Aunt Lou. Years ago I had been fond of her; she had been warmer than the other aunts, less talky and vicious, and during the first years when Donald was away in New York, she had visited my mother often. She was fun to talk with, and she loved going shopping and having dinner out. I thought she had escaped the family malady of neurosis. But in time she, like my mother, my aunt Etta, and two uncles, was sucked down into dementia. Now she was killing Donald.

"Well," I said to Donald lamely, "try to take care of yourself."

He gave a bitter little chuckle as if I'd told a painful joke. "How's Manny?" he asked, and I knew he was about to end the conversation.

"Well—not so good. His feet have swollen so he can hardly stand, even to go to the bathroom. I think it's from sitting in the wheelchair day in and day out."

"Too bad. He still living by himself?" Manny had chosen to continue living in our parents' house. He wasn't asking me or anyone else to take care of him.

"He's got a couple of roomers who help in a lot of ways. You know, taking out the trash and stuff. But I don't know how much longer he can make it like that."

We talked for a little while longer. Then Donald said something that later struck me as strange, at least for him: "Sometimes I wonder why God does some things. Sister Little, do you believe in God?"

I was taken aback. We had never talked about religion, and I felt shy and uncomfortable. "Well, yeah, sure."

"Me, too. I don't understand Him, but I believe."

Something led me to say what I'd never said to him before. The words didn't come easy. "I love you."

And he replied, "I love you."

That was all we said, but I have thought of that exchange many times since.

A few weeks later he called to say he had put Aunt Lou in a nursing home. By now she was unaware where she was. She spent all her hours in a deep slumber, her hands tied to the bed so that she could not disturb the tubes that connected her wasted body to life. Now and then she called out for Donald. He was always there.

I told him that I was glad she was finally in a home. Maybe now he would get some rest.

Another four A.M. hell. Sitting here staring at this canvas since midnight, but no picture comes. Brush damp where I've been clutching it, easel ready. No picture. All these thoughts whirling around in my head. But no picture. House too quiet. Lost in all that silence. Quiet like death. No picture. Pee dark again

like mud. Everything hurts. Call Gladys when it gets light. Ask her take me to the hospital when she goes see Horace. Drop me off at Emergency. I'm dying and I know it.

The family was shocked. Those who had berated him for putting his mother "away" were, for a time, silenced. Nobody had thought he was really sick. Nobody had thought of him in any way except as Aunt Lou's caregiver. They felt tricked because he had died before her. The whisper went around the mortuary, even as the wake began, that Donald had died of AIDS. Those who had called him a sissy felt vindicated.

As for me, looking down at him through tears, I wondered that none of us, myself most of all, had seen how pale and thin he had become, and how the crinkly sandy-white hair was gone and his head was covered with a cheap brown wig. Why don't we look at one another until one leans over the other's coffin?

I gasped at the force of the pain that flashed through me. Why didn't I know? Why didn't he tell me? I heard again whispers of conversations: ". . . if I can get someone to stay with Lou . . ." (and I never said, "I'll stay.") ". . . my stomach stays upset and my back pains me . . ." ". . . liver infection . . ." "Sister Little, do you believe in God?" And all the things we never talked about. The loneliness of his living in a world primarily heterosexual. A whole side of him that I pretended didn't exist. I used to tell myself that it didn't matter that he was gay. But it should have mattered. Because that's who he was. The most important, intimate side of him, his whole life style, invisible because I wouldn't see.

I had thought we were close, but he had endured alone his pain and the terrible knowledge of impending death.

As I stood there, his face still blurred by my tears, incongruously I remembered a painting that I had seen in a book somewhere years ago. A hooded figure stood before a closed door wreathed by weeds, rank and thick. The door had no knob. On it, in letters barely legible, were scrawled the saddest of words: *That which I should have done I did not do.* And I wept.

Aunt Lou is still vegetating in Holy Light Nursing Home. Now and then she still rouses and mutters something that sounds like, "Donald! Donald!" Then she sinks back into slumber.

30

Atlantis

✑ *Mark Doty*

I. FAITH

"I've been having these
awful dreams, each a little different,
though the core's the same—

we're walking in a field,
Wally and Arden and I, a stretch of grass
with a highway running beside it,

or a path in the woods that opens
onto a road. Everything's fine,
then the dog sprints ahead of us,

excited; we're calling but
he's racing down a scent and doesn't hear us,
and that's when he goes

onto the highway. I don't want to describe it.
Sometimes it's brutal and over,
and others he's struck and takes off

so we don't know where he is
or how bad. This wakes me
every night now, and I stay awake;

I'm afraid if I sleep I'll go back
into the dream. It's been six months,
almost exactly, since the doctor wrote

not even a real word
but an acronym, a vacant
four-letter cipher

that draws meanings into itself,
reconstitutes the world.
We tried to say it was just

a word; we tried to admit
it had power and thus to nullify it
by means of our acknowledgement.

I know the current wisdom:
bright hope, the power of wishing you're well.
He's just so tired, though nothing

shows in any tests, Nothing,
the doctor says, detectable;
the doctor doesn't hear what I do,

that trickling, steadily rising nothing
that makes him sleep all day,
vanish into fever's tranced afternoons,

and I swear sometimes
when I put my head to his chest
I can hear the virus humming

like a refrigerator.
Which is what makes me think
you can take your positive attitude

and go straight to hell.
We don't have a future,
we have a dog.
    Who is he?

Soul without speech,
sheer, tireless faith,
he is that-which-goes-forward,

black muzzle, black paws
scouting what's ahead;
he is where we'll be hit first,

he's the part of us
that's going to get it.
I'm hardly awake on our morning walk

—always just me and Arden now—
and sometimes I am still
in the thrall of the dream,

which is why, when he took a step onto Commercial
before I'd looked both ways,
I screamed his name and grabbed his collar.

And there I was on my knees,
both arms around his neck
and nothing coming,

and when I looked into that bewildered face
I realized I didn't know what it was
I was shouting at,

I didn't know who I was trying to protect."

2. REPRIEVE

I woke in the night
and thought, *It was a dream,*

nothing has torn the future apart,
we have not lived years

in dread, it never happened,
I dreamed it all. And then

there was this sensation of terrific pressure
lifting, as if I were rising

in one of those old diving bells,
lightening, unburdening. I didn't know

how heavy my life had become—so much fear,
so little knowledge. It was like

being young again, but I understood
how light I was, how without encumbrance,—

and so I felt both young and awake,
which I never felt

when I *was* young. The curtains moved
—it was still summer, all the windows open—

and I thought, I can move that easily.
I thought my dream had lasted for years,

a decade, a dream can seem like that,
I thought, *There's so much more time . . .*

And then of course the truth
came floating back to me.

You know how children
love to end stories they tell

by saying, It was all a dream? Years ago,
when I taught kids to write,

I used to tell them this ending spoiled things,
explaining and dismissing

what had come before. Now I know
how wise they were, to prefer

that gesture of closure,
their stories rounded not with a sleep

but a waking. What other gift
comes close to a reprieve?

This was the dream that Wally told me:
I was in the tunnel, he said,

and there really was a light at the end,
and a great being standing in the light.

His arms were full of people, men and women,
but his proportions were all just right—I mean

he was the size of you or me.
And the people said, Come with us,

we're going dancing. And they seemed so glad
to be going, and so glad to have me

join them, but I said,
I'm not ready yet. I didn't know what to do,

when he finished,
except hold the relentless

weight of him, I didn't know
what to say except, *It was a dream,*

nothing's wrong now,
it was only a dream.

3. MICHAEL'S DREAM

Michael writes to tell me his dream:
I was helping Randy out of bed,
supporting him on one side
with another friend on the other,

and as we stood him up, he stepped out
of the body I was holding and became
a shining body, brilliant light
held in the form I first knew him in.

This is what I imagine will happen,
the spirit's release. Michael,
when we support our friends,
one of us on either side, our arms

under the man or woman's arms,
what is it we're holding? Vessel,
shadow, hurrying light? All those years
I made love to a man without thinking

how little his body had to do with me;
now, diminished, he's never been so plainly
himself—remote and unguarded,
an otherness I can't know

the first thing about. I said,
You need to drink more water
or you're going to turn into
an old dry leaf. And he said,

Maybe I want to be an old leaf.
In the dream Randy's leaping into
the future, and still here; Michael's holding him
and releasing at once. Just as Steve's

holding Jerry, though he's already gone,
Marie holding John, gone, Maggie holding
her John, gone, Carlos and Darren
holding another Michael, gone,

and I'm holding Wally, who's going.
Where isn't the question,
though we think it is;
we don't even know where the living are,

in this raddled and unraveling "here."
What is the body? Rain on a window,
a clear movement over whose gaze?
Husk, leaf, little boat of paper

and wood to mark the speed of the stream?
Randy and Jerry, Michael and Wally

and John: lucky we don't have to know
what something is in order to hold it.

4. ATLANTIS

I thought your illness a kind of solvent
dissolving the future a little at a time;

I didn't understand what's to come
was always just a glimmer

up ahead, veiled like the marsh
gone under its tidal sheet

of mildly rippling aluminum.
What these salt distances were

is also where they're going:
from blankly silvered span

toward specificity: the curve
of certain brave islands of grass,

temporary shoulder-wide rivers
where herons ply their twin trades

of study and desire. I've seen
two white emissaries unfold

like heaven's linen, untouched,
enormous, a fluid exhalation. Early spring,

too cold yet for green, too early
for the tumble and wrack of last season

to be anything but promise,
but there in the air was white tulip,

marvel, triumph of all flowering, the soul
lifted up, if we could still believe

in the soul, after so much diminishment . . .
Breath, from the unpromising waters,

up, across the pond and the two-lane highway,
pure purpose, over the dune,

gone. Tomorrow's unreadable
as this shining acreage;

the future's nothing
but this moment's gleaming rim.

Now the tide's begun
its clockwork turn, pouring,

in the day's hourglass,
toward the other side of the world,

and our dependable marsh reappears
—emptied of that starched and angular grace

that spirited the ether, lessened,
but here. And our ongoingness,

what there'll be of us? Look,
love, the lost world

rising from the waters again:
our continent, where it always was,

emerging from the half-light, unforgettable,
drenched, unchanged.

5. COASTAL

Cold April and the neighbor girl
   —our plumber's daughter—
      comes up the wet street

from the harbor carrying,
   in a nest she's made
      of her pink parka,

a loon. It's so sick,
　　she says when I ask.
　　　　Foolish kid,

does she think she can keep
　　this emissary of air?
　　　　Is it trust or illness

that allows the head
　　—sleek tulip—to bow
　　　　on its bent stem

across her arm?
　　Look at the steady,
　　　　quiet eye. She is carrying

the bird back from indifference,
　　from the coast
　　　　of whatever rearrangement

the elements intend,
　　and the loon allows her.
　　　　She is going to call

the Center for Coastal Studies,
　　and will swaddle the bird
　　　　in her petal-bright coat

until they come.
　　She cradles the wild form.
　　　　Stubborn girl.

6. NEW DOG

Jimi and Tony
can't keep Dino,
their cocker spaniel;
Tony's too sick,
the daily walks
more pressure
than pleasure,

one more obligation
that can't be met.

And though we already
have a dog, Wally
wants to adopt,
wants something small
and golden to sleep
next to him and
lick his face.
He's paralyzed now
from the waist down,

whatever's ruining him
moving upward, and
we don't know
how much longer
he'll be able to pet
a dog. How many men
want another attachment,
just as they're
leaving the world?

Wally sits up nights
and says, *I'd like
some lizards, a talking bird,
some fish. A little rat.*

So after I drive
to Jimi and Tony's
in the Village and they
meet me at the door and say,
We can't go through with it,

we can't give up our dog,
I drive to the shelter
—just to look—and there
is Beau: bounding and
practically boundless,
one brass concatenation
of tongue and tail,

unmediated energy,
too big, wild,

perfect. He not only
licks Wally's face
but bathes every
irreplaceable inch
of his head, and though
Wally can no longer
feed himself he can lift
his hand, and bring it
to rest on the rough gilt

flanks when they are,
for a moment, still.
I have never seen a touch
so deliberate.
It isn't about grasping;
the hand itself seems
almost blurred now,
softened, though
tentative only

because so much will
must be summoned,
such attention brought
to the work—which is all
he is now, this gesture
toward the restless splendor,
the unruly, the golden,
the animal, the new.

31

Oceanic Hotel, Nice

Tereze Glück

Nicholas said, "I must have a cigarette."

Said is not exactly accurate, since he could hardly speak. It was, I think, a matter of strength, or lack of it—he just did not have the strength to use his voice. He whispered, kind of. To hear him I had to lean over, so that my ear was near his mouth. I hated this. His breath was warm and sour-smelling. I was as squeamish as a startled cat that starts at any sound, and slinks away, its body low to the ground, as if it thinks no one can see it. I thought germs were coming towards me on his breath—viruses like rain. His breath was hot, and also moist. I hated everything.

"The Chapel," Nicholas said.

"The Chapel?"

"I must have a cigarette," he said.

I looked at him dumbly.

"My pants," he said. All of this in that half-whisper.

"What?" I said.

He tried to gesture. He could not gesture any better than he could speak. This gesture consisted of a raised forefinger. I tried to follow some logical line of direction. I turned around and saw the closet, and a pair of sweatpants shoved onto the shelf.

Surely, I said to myself, surely he does not expect me to put these on him? Because it was clear he could not put them on himself. He could not so much as lift his arm, never mind his leg.

I got the sweatpants down from the closet. "I'll get a nurse," I said. This seemed a little shameful. But I was more relieved than ashamed.

I turned my back while they pulled the sweatpants over his legs. His legs were—you know. As thin as everything you remember—the prisoners of war at Andersonville, those famous photographs, or the survivors at the concentration camps. I am not exaggerating. I am not making one of those venal comparisons—you know, this or that is like the Holocaust. I am simply describing his legs, and the best description is in these images. There was almost nothing left of his legs. They were bones with skin pulled over them. There was no calf to speak of.

"Can you put him in the wheelchair?" I said to the nurse. I was thinking, Bless these people, I can't believe they do what they do. I was as nervous as a cat. I wanted just to get out of there. The whole place smelled of illness with an overlay of soursweet camouflage. Hospitals don't smell spanking clean—of Clorox, or laundry, or bright bleached things—they smell of illness and the effort to mask it. The smell can make you sick. When I am in a hospital I try not to breathe too deeply.

"My sweater," Nicholas said.

The sweater was on a chair. I was as afraid of the sweater as I was of him. The sweater was dirty, with stains on it that maybe were food and maybe were blood as well. The sweater was matted. Under my fingers the sweater felt like old foul things dried and caked over. Nicholas's whole apartment was like that, until one Saturday Gwen and I just went to clean it up. We went to Woolworth's and bought every cleaning supply you could think of and rubber gloves. I said, "I'd just like to hose this place down." Gwen says I repeated this many times during the course of that day. We went there when we thought Nicholas was in Paris, only it turned out he wasn't in Paris at all, he was in the hospital, but we didn't know that. He did make it to Paris, apparently, but he collapsed there, or had a seizure, or something, and was taken to the hospital in Paris and the next day was somehow put on an airplane for New York and was met at the airport by some friends, not us, other friends, and was taken to a hospital in New York. That was last fall, and it was spring now; that was a different hospital stay, a different episode, although when I think back on it, it may be more accurate to say that it was just the beginning of a long episode which seemed to be shaping up to be, well, his last. Since then he never really got back home for more than a few days before landing in the hospital again.

To put the sweater on him I had to touch his arm, which made me feel faint.

"Oh dear," I said to him. "I'm afraid I'm no caretaker." I smiled. I got one arm in an armhole and somehow managed to get the sweater behind him and his other arm in. I felt faint again—I mean exactly that, as if I would faint. I lectured myself. If it's awful to be *near* this, I said, imagine what it's like to *be* this. But in truth this meant nothing to me—my whole body replied, But I am *not* this! This is *not* happening to me and I'm glad it's not! This was said in protest. This was physical health resenting the tyranny of illness. This was one self encountering the fact that it was not in fact another self. This was me being imperial.

Still the sweater got on him somehow. The sick feeling in my stomach did not go away. Now we had to get him into the wheelchair. All this had taken, fifteen, twenty minutes. All this for a cigarette.

A cigarette, of course, was pretty much all that was left to him.

I went out to the nurse's station. "Could somebody put Mr. Rhodes in a wheelchair please?"

"Where you taking him?" a young man said.

"To the Chapel," I said.

The nurses had a discussion about who would do it. The one who was on duty was eating a sandwich. "It's my lunch hour," she said. Another one said, "That's all right, you eat, I'll do it." This impressed me. This was the kind of helpful behavior we are led to believe has died out, but imagine, here it was, and right in the heart of New York City.

There was some discussion between the nurse and the young male nurse about how to best get Nicholas out of the bed and into the wheelchair. As experienced as they were, they were still perplexed. Finally they swung Nicholas's legs from the bed so that his feet dangled over the side of the bed. Then they lifted his shoulders and swung his body kind of sideways. I'm not sure what they did next; I think I turned and walked out into the hall. When I turned back around he was already in the chair. His face was gaunt and exhausted. He looked to me like one of those portraits of Christ, where Christ can't hold up his head, and his head leans to one side, and his entire body is limp with suffering. The male nurse came up to us. "Now Mr. Rhodes," he said. "No little side trips, you hear? No little side stops for a cigarette or anything like that." Then he turned to me, as if neither of us could hear what was addressed to the other. "You take him to the Chapel and that's it," he said. "No little side trips for cigarettes. Okay?"

I stared dumbly at the young man. "Well," I said.

"No cigarettes," he said. "This is a no-smoking hospital."

"Look," I said. "You be the one to tell him, not me."

He knelt and spoke to Nicholas. "No cigarettes Mr. Rhodes, you got that? This is a no-smoking hospital and that's the rule. It's not fair to other patients."

Then he turned back to me. He seemed to want some kind of answer, which was difficult, because I never could lie, not even small lies about unimportant things. I hung my head like an errant child. Then I looked up at him. I had the feeling that I had a kind of pleading look on my face. "Look," I said. "What difference does it make if he smokes or not? For God's sake, it's his only pleasure. Can't he just have a cigarette? Who does it hurt?"

The male nurse looked at me. "I sympathize," he said. "Believe me, I'm a smoker myself. But those are the rules."

I shook my head. I was trying to work myself up to the required lie.

"Look," the man said. "Just don't tell me. That's all. Just don't tell me."

"Which way's the Chapel?" I said, looking him in the eye.

It took a few minutes to get down to the Chapel. I wasn't very spry with a wheelchair. Nicholas's feet kept dragging, and he didn't have the strength to lift them onto the footrests of the wheelchair, and I didn't want to touch them. Every now and then I'd stop and try to lift his feet anyway, which made me shudder. All this time I was just thinking what a bad person I was to not even want to touch his feet, but there it was—I just didn't, it made me shudder, and that's that. He had on those thin stretch foam slippers they give you in hospitals, and the slippers kept coming off his heels, so that they hung from his toes. I'd stop the wheelchair and squat down and try to pull the slippers on without actually having to touch his skin, and then I'd try to lift his legs by just holding on to the slippers. In fact I did not succeed, not with the slippers or the footrest, and we'd wheel along and I'd hear his feet dragging along the floor.

Just as we got to the Chapel a man came in with a woman and a child. The man had an IV hooked up to him and wore the blue robe of the hospital. He had bandages around his head. He sat down in the back with the woman and the child. "Fuck" said Nicholas. Of all the things he had said to me today this was the clearest.

"I'm sure they won't stay long," I said. After all, it wasn't as if *he* wanted a cigarette, which could take some time if you wanted to enjoy a few. He was only here to talk to God, presumably, and let's face it, conversations with God are pretty one-sided and after the first few minutes all you do is start to repeat yourself. I figure I'm as qualified to speak about this as the next fellow. I talked to God endlessly and I was always saying the same thing. I read a lot of self-help books which explained to me that I was doing the wrong kind of praying, which I had always somehow known, my idea of a prayer being to really really really beg God for whatever it was I wanted. When I didn't get it, which I never did, I always thought it was because I hadn't wanted it hard enough and the thing to do was want it *more.* As dialogues with God go, I'd have to admit that mine were pretty primitive, not to mention missing the point, so it wasn't altogether surprising that my prayers were never answered.

Although maybe they were answered only who could decipher the answer? Which was always the problem with God in the first place.

After a few minutes, the man in the Chapel got up and left, followed by his IV rigging, the woman and the child. "Thank bloody God," Nicholas said.

He tried to get his cigarettes but he really couldn't move his arm, so I got them for him, gingerly, the way I'd put his slippers back on his feet. The sweater was, frankly, a mess. God knows what was on that sweater. I hated to think what was on that sweater.

I had some reasons to shudder in the matter of the sweater. Last fall my friend Gwen and I had gone to Nicholas's apartment to clean it up. It was so foul, so dirty, I couldn't bear to go there. When Nicholas and I would make a date, he'd say, "Meet me at my apartment and we'll have a little drink," and finally I said to him, "Nicholas, I just can't go to your apartment any more." This may sound extreme but then, his apartment was something extreme. So we would meet in restaurants.

All this was before he was in the hospital, when he could still get around some, could still go out to a restaurant for dinner. He was planning a trip to Paris—in retrospect this seems sheer madness, he was so ill, but he had got as far as he had got precisely by imagining trips to Paris and then *taking* them, God damn it. For some time he'd been living mostly on will, and it wasn't a halfbad program at that. So he went to Paris, and Gwen and I decided to clean his apartment while he was gone as a surprise for him. Really I did it for myself because the apartment just made me so outright sick I couldn't stand it. I just wanted to clean the God-damned thing. I just wanted to *hose* the God-damned place down. A good hosing down was exactly what it needed. I don't want to elaborate, but that apartment was thick with things you wouldn't believe—caked blood on the mouthpiece of the telephone and on the sheets, and thick layers of oozy substances that had dried. Some of them were food and some of them, well, weren't. The sheets were filled with cigarette holes with charred edges. Gwen said, It's amazing he never set fire to himself.

We put on rubber gloves and just went at it. Our original plan was to hire someone to do it and we'd just kind of oversee the task, and in fact we did hire someone, but when she started in cleaning Gwen and I looked at each other and just pitched in. Gwen said later, when we were having a drink and congratulating ourselves, Well we couldn't exactly just stand there and watch her clean. In the end it took three of us all day and we didn't even finish at that. The woman we hired, whose name was Marilyn and who was very kind, something you could just tell about her right off, cleaned the kitchen and the bathroom, and Gwen and I did the living room and the bedroom. There was a little study and in fact we never even got to the study and to tell the truth, one day was enough. One day could make you feel like a saint, which we did.

We found two dead mice under a fine mahogany table in the living room.

Also, we threw out all the bedclothes.

So I had some reason to be fearful of the sweater. But everything I was doing was something I hated, so I just grimaced and did this as well—put my hand in the pocket of his sweater and got his cigarettes. I took one out and put it between his lips.

"Water," Nicholas said.

"What about water?" I said.

"Get some water. For the ashes," he said.

"But I don't have a cup or anything. Where do I get water?"

"Go look for a kitchen or something."

"Look you can just tip your ashes onto the carpet. They're good for the carpet." I remembered how, when we were in college, everyone always used to say that. Everyone used to drop their ashes onto the carpet and rub them into the carpet with their feet and shrug and say, "It's good for the carpet."

But he was insistent so I left him there, with the organ and the pews and the stained glass windows, and went to find a water fountain, and a cup to put the water in. I found the fountain but no cup. I kept wandering until I saw some people in uniforms—orderlies, maybe, something like that—and I stopped them and said "Excuse me, where can I get a cup? Is there a kitchen on this floor or something?" but they just shrugged and said no, there wasn't. When I'd been gone a few minutes I thought I just better get back to Nicholas. He'd just have to use the floor, that was all.

So I went back to the Chapel. He was still there, slumped in his wheel-chair. I'd been half-afraid I'd find him on the floor.

"I couldn't find a cup anywhere," I said. "Just use the floor. It's good for the carpet."

"What about the stub?" he said.

There was a fire exit right near us, that opened onto an alleylike affair. "The fire exit," I said. Then I got half-afraid I'd put the stub out and get myself locked out in the alley. I had a whole, instant daydream about this—like something out of the old Alfred Hitchcock Television Hour they used to show on Sunday nights when I was growing up—I'd be locked out on this landing that didn't go anywhere, and Nicholas would be in his wheel-chair, unable to open the door, unable to call out for help.

"Matches," Nicholas whispered.

I looked in the cigarette box, and fished around again in the pocket of his sweater, and then the other pocket. There were no matches.

"Nicholas, there are no matches," I said. I felt oddly relieved, as if fate had taken over and it was all out of my hands. Everything would be over more quickly now, if he couldn't have his cigarette, and then I'd be able to get out of there. Get out of there and go home, and wash my hands, and have a hot bath.

"Oh God," Nicholas said. "Can't you go find matches?" he said.

"But who could I ask?" I said. "You're not supposed to be smoking."

"Look," I said. "I think we just better forget the cigarette thing."

I wheeled him out of the Chapel and down the hall toward the elevator. It was all the way at the other end of the floor, so it took a few minutes. Nicholas's feet dragged along the floor, and his slippers kept slipping off his heels. Every now and then I stopped and tried to put them back on and tried to put his feet up on the footrest, but I wasn't doing any better than I'd done before.

We waited for the elevator. Hospital elevators always seem to take forever, and this one was.

When it came, it had a lot of people in it, and they had to move to make room for the wheelchair. I wheeled Nicholas in and he said to a man next to him, almost as clearly as he'd said the word "Fuck" earlier when he saw the man in the Chapel, "Excuse me but do you have any matches?" The man put his hand in his pocket and like a magician pulled out a book of matches. I just laughed and laughed.

So we rode back down in the elevator and went back to the Chapel. "God damn it Nicholas," I said, laughing. "Nothing like a little motivation." This was why he was still alive at all.

We went through the whole thing again. I got the cigarettes out of his pocket, and put one between his dried cracked lips, and lit a match. He managed to hold the cigarette in his hands, holding onto it as if it were something that could support his weight, something he could lean against. But he couldn't tip his ashes. When the ash got long, I'd take the cigarette and tap it, and the ashes fell onto the floor, and I rubbed them into the carpet with my foot.

When it was time to put out the stub I opened the fire door, and I had my daydream again. I was careful to hold the door open when I ground out the stub on the cement.

Then we did it all again.

All in all Nicholas smoked three cigarettes. He sighed. "I haven't had a cigarette in four days," he said. Not since his last visitor.

After the third cigarette I said I had to go. I took him back upstairs and the nurses took him out of the wheelchair and put him back into the bed. We said good-bye and I rode the elevator down to the main lobby. I was walking out the door to the street and there was a woman walking out the door right beside me, and I said to her, "I hate hospitals, I just hate them. If anything ever happens to me I swear I'll just *die* before I end up in one of these places." I was outright shuddering. She looked at me as if I were very strange. "Really?" she said.

I walked up Seventh Avenue and stopped at Barney's. I spent an hour there, and I bought something expensive. I was trying to get the hospital out of my head, and its smell off my skin. I was trying to replace the hospital with aesthetic pleasure, expense, silk, perfume, gold jewelry, fine linen.

We had some fine old times together, Nicholas and I. We found each other very funny, very clever. We made each other laugh and were pleased with ourselves. Also we both liked good things—fine meals, good champagne, expensive clothes. We had some extraordinary meals, and not just in New York. We had them in Rome, and in Positano and Capri, and a couple of years later in Paris. We were once at a famous restaurant in Rome, although I forget its name even if it was famous. Nicholas would remember its name. He knew the names of all the best restaurants in Rome and Paris. It was early evening and we were sitting outdoors among a long row of tables. We were feeling very jolly, very witty. We were with a couple of other people, so we made a lively group. Someone said something, it doesn't matter what, and we all laughed loudly. A man at the table behind us said, Well you'd *think* they could keep their *voices* down. He was with a boyfriend, that much was clear. They were Americans. We laughed again, over something else, and the man said, very uppity-like, directly to us this time, Could you *please* keep your voices down? We just shrugged and he said Hmph, you could at *least* be *polite*. Nicholas was smoking a cigarette and he turned around and smiled and said, "Oh, but we couldn't *possibly*."

That was when he had money, before he had to pay all his money to his doctors and for medicine. He was independently wealthy, he had always been a rich boy, so of course he had no insurance. What was there to be afraid of in those days? He got some venereal diseases, which was just par for the course, his course anyway, and he got an inconvenient abscess which ended up restricting his sex life somewhat, but why did he have to worry about insurance? He was young and essentially healthy and rich, and even more than that, he was talented. He wrote two books and published them to some fine reviews. So when he got sick he had to use all his money for his treatments. Then he had no more money so he went on welfare and was a ward of the state. Even then we kept going out to good restaurants. He had an apartment in Paris, from the days when he was rich, and got some money from renting it. He didn't get enough to live on, never mind enough to pay for his medicines, but he got some, and what he got he used for dinners out, when he could still go out.

The last time we had dinner together was in the fall, just before the trip to Paris when Gwen and I cleaned his apartment. I met him at his apartment even though I hated going there. I wouldn't have a drink, though. This bothered him but it wasn't just the disease, it was the filth in the apartment. I told him this outright. I wasn't about to lie to him. Maybe I should have, but then, I couldn't even lie to an orderly in a hospital about a cigarette.

His apartment was on the third floor of a townhouse, and there was no elevator. I went down the stairs first. I didn't help him because it was easier for him to hold on to the bannister than to me. He could hardly walk. The disease had done something to his feet, I wasn't sure what. He had neuropathy, although I'm not sure if that's what made for the difficulty in walking. In any case he could no longer walk very well. He was very skinny and weak. I waited at the bottom of the stairs. Every now and then he'd curse. We went down the front stoop to the sidewalk. Nicholas held on to the railing of the stone steps while I hailed a cab. He started toward the curb, to the cab, but when he walked he would trip over his feet—one foot would somehow end up a little in front of the other, so that when he took the next step his foot would be in his way. He tripped and grabbed hold of the railing, which was still within reach. "Fuck," he said. I went to help him, and put my arm through his, but I was shuddering.

It took us so long to get to the restaurant that when we got there, they had given our table away. I'd booked a table in the smoking section of course, so Nicholas could smoke, but they had to seat us in non-smoking. Every time he wanted a cigarette he had to go over to the bar. It took him forever to walk to the bar, so I spent a lot of the dinner sitting alone at the table, waiting for him.

The food was good; I remember. A restaurant critic was at a table nearby. Various people whispered her name and glanced over at her table. Nicholas and I sat next to a very nice young man and woman. I don't know if they were a couple or if they were just friends. We fell into conversation with them and it turned out her brother had died of AIDS. She was very friendly, very forthcoming. In fact when Nicholas wanted a cigarette she walked with him to the bar. She was being much nicer to him than I was. For me this was the beginning of the decline—I think of it that way—in which his presence, formerly a pleasure, had become a burden. *He* hadn't given up but it seemed that *I* had.

We weren't making clever conversation any more. We were trying, but trying only made it worse. There is something truly awful about bravery, I find. It makes you kind of weak in the stomach. Give me misery any day. At least it's honest.

Nicholas's teeth had fallen out long ago. He'd had false teeth made, but they were a problem. They were one of the reasons we'd been so late for dinner and had lost our table. It took him a long time to put them in. While I waited for him in the living room of his apartment, I could hear him cursing in the bathroom while he tried to put his teeth in. I guess they weren't very comfortable, because it wasn't easy for him to eat. I was sitting across from him, at this wonderful restaurant, where the food was inventive and elaborately presented, so I couldn't help but see him, the gingerish, painstaking way he'd eat. He would drool a little, bits of food would fall down his chin. He still made a great ritual of offering me a taste of his food, and sometimes I would take a little from his plate before he began to eat, and I always gave him some of mine to taste, but in fact I had come to hate the ritual, its insistence, its provocation and denial. He was doing something for himself with this ritual—making claim to some normalcy, and making a statement—but I was reduced to audience, a functionary of his gesture. I tried to hold up my end, but I was minding more and more, and the fact is I was no good at dissembling.

That night, when I sat looking across the table at him, I kept thinking: Let me out of here, let me out of here.

I just wanted to run away.

I was as miserable as a sick cat. I could hardly make myself smile.

I took him home, and he held my arm as we walked toward his front stoop. I turned to look at him while he was talking and I said, "Nicholas, you're bleeding." His mouth was bleeding. He stopped and found a handkerchief and held it to his mouth.

I took him upstairs and got a cab for myself. When I got in the cab I saw that there was blood on my sleeve. I sat with my arm held away from me, as far as I could get it. I was shuddering as if I could shake it off—I mean the arm, or the blood. Shuddering was getting to be my main mode, at least so far as Nicholas was concerned.

When I got to my apartment I found a pair of rubber gloves under the sink and I put them on. I took my coat off and hung it on the door of the closet, away from anything else. I went into my daughter's room. The room was dark and she was asleep. "You took sex education, didn't you?" I said in a loud whisper. There is something about the dark that makes us whisper, even when it's our intention to wake somebody up.

She bolted up in the bed. "What?" she said.

"You took sex education, right?"

"Why?" she said.

"I got Nicholas's blood on my coat," I said. "I can't get sick from that, can I? I mean—you took sex education; you'd know, right?"

"Mother, I need to sleep," she said.

In the morning I took the coat to the cleaners, and I've worn it often since then. I say that as if to acquit myself of something—some mean and furtive criminal act, such as fear.

Shortly after that Nicholas left for Paris and Gwen and I went down to clean his apartment, only of course he wasn't in Paris very long at all, and at the time Gwen and I were cleaning his apartment he was already in

St. Vincent's Hospital, only no one had told us. Eventually I located him, and went to see him in the hospital, where he said to me, "I must have a cigarette."

I would say my decline was complete by then.

After the hospital, when I got to Barney's, I smelled the perfumes, and looked over the china and glassware, and I even tried on some expensive clothing I knew I would never buy. I tried on a black dress made out of the same fabric they use for tuxedos, and I was looking at myself in the mirror. I just stood there and stared at myself. I stared and I said to myself, "You have no compassion." This was uttered coolly, just a cool assessment, an objective remark as neutral as a comment about the color of my eyes or the length of my hair. It was just a fact, like any other fact—trees, sky, concrete, illness, death. In the mirror, through the fine fabric of the black dress, it was as if I could see a burned-out center in the middle of my body, where a heart used to beat; and even this failed to move me. Upon reflection this is not so surprising; for, what was left to be moved?

I did not buy the black dress. It was too expensive, and in any case I had no place to wear it. I went back down to the main floor and bought a lemony perfume called "Oceanic Hotel Nice." The bottle had an art deco picture on it, in bright blue and a mustard yellow, of a boulevard with a palm tree and the facade of a hotel. It could very well be Nice. I'd been there once, some years ago. It was raining when we were there, and we did not stay for long, but I bought a tin of olive oil, for which Nice was famous if I am not mistaken. I still have it, somewhere in the back of a kitchen shelf, unopened I expect. I'm like that—I buy things and then I forget to use them. But I wear this perfume all the time; it's my offering. Of course Nicholas would have preferred a cigarette, but I don't get downtown often.

PART V
Paid Caregivers

Caregiving is such a big job that many family members cannot do it on their own. The people they hire or who are sent by agencies because the patient is entitled to this service become essential complements to the care the family provides. This relationship is often fraught with ambiguity. These paid caregivers are not "family" in the traditional, or even nontraditional, sense; they are employees. Yet they become integrated into the routines and problems of daily life. These stories illustrate some of the complications that occur. They also portray these workers as individuals with different personalities and beliefs, not as interchangeable helpers.

In "A Pension Plan" by Ha Jin, Jufen is the home care aide who takes care of Mr. Sheng, who suffers from dementia. She performs the daily routine of personal care and taking him out for walks. The plot revolves around Minna, Mr. Sheng's daughter, who first fires Jufen and then asks that she return with a proposal that shocks the aide into thinking about her own future.

The only selection in this volume set in an assisted living facility, "A Bad Day for Pisces" by Fran Pokras Yariv, is narrated by Ofelia, an aide in the Sunset Hills Retirement Community. On the good side of the ledger is her fondness for her client, Mrs. Breur. On the bad side is her difficulty with her client's daughter, Ms. Breur-Gordon.

In "Wheelchair" by Lewis Nordan, Harris, the paid attendant, appears only in the final pages, yet he is crucial to the story. It is his absence that Winston Krepps, the person in the wheelchair, deplores. Harris has not returned from his day off, and Winston is left to navigate on his own. His struggles are described in all their clinical detail. Yet he is not angry at Harris, he just wants him there.

"God's Goodness," by Marjorie Kemper, is the story of Ling Tan, an aide who is sent to help Mike, a sixteen-year-old boy who is dying. Ling lives with Mike and his mother, Mrs. Tipton. Ling and Mike carry on a dialogue about hope and miracles and the Book of Job. Ling's experience challenges her Christian faith in the power of prayer.

32

A Pension Plan

& *Ha Jin*

It was said that Mr. Sheng suffered from a kind of senile dementia caused by
some infarction in his brain. I was sure it was neither Parkinson's nor Alzheimer's, because I had learned quite a bit about both during my training to
be a health aide. He wasn't completely disabled, but he needed to be cared
for during the day. I was glad to attend to him, because I'd been out of work
for more than three months before this job.

Every morning I'd wash his face with a hand towel soaked with warm
water, but I'd been told I mustn't shave him, which only his family members
could do. He was sixty-nine, gentle by nature and soft-spoken. He'd taught
physics at a middle school back in Changchun City three decades ago, but
he couldn't read his old textbooks anymore and was unable to remember the
formulas and the theorems. He still could recognize many words, though.
He often had a newspaper on his lap when sitting alone. My job was to cook
for him, feed him, keep him clean, and take him around. A young nurse
came every other day to check his vital signs and give him an injection. The
twentysomething told me that actually there was no cure for Mr. Sheng's
illness, which the doctor could only try to keep under control and slow down
his deterioration. I felt lucky that my charge wasn't violent like many victims
of dementia.

Mr. Sheng's wife had died long ago, before he came to the United States,
but he believed she was still alive. Oftentimes he couldn't remember her
name, so every morning I let him look through an album that contained
about two dozen photos of her and him together. In the pictures, they were
young and appeared to be a happy couple. She was a pretty woman, the kind
of beauty with glossy skin and a delicate figure you often find in the prov-
inces south of the Yangtze River. Sometimes when I pointed at her face and
asked him, "Who's this?" he'd raise his eyes and look at me, his face blank.

About a month after I started, his daughter, Minna, intervened, saying the photos might upset him and I shouldn't show them to him anymore, so I put the album away. He never complained about its absence. Minna was a little bossy, but I didn't mind. She must have loved her dad. She called me Aunt Niu. That made me uneasy, because I had just turned forty-eight, not that old.

Part of my job was to feed Mr. Sheng. I often had to cajole him into swallowing food. Sometimes he was like a sick baby who refused to hold food in its mouth for long. I made fine meals for him—chicken porridge, fish dumplings, shrimp and taro pottage, noodles mixed with shredded shiitake mushrooms, but in spite of his full set of teeth, he seemed unable to tell any difference among most of the foods. A good part of his taste buds must have been dead. When eating, he'd jabber between mouthfuls, his words by and large incomprehensible. Yet once in a while he'd pause to ask me, "See what I mean?"

I'd keep mute. If pressed further, I'd shake my head and admit, "No, I didn't follow you."

"You always space out," he'd grunt, then refuse to eat any more.

Lunch usually took more than two hours. That didn't bother me, since in essence my job was just to help him while away time. Due to his willfulness about food, I decided to eat my own meal before feeding him.

After lunch we often went out for some fresh air, to do a little shopping and get that day's World Journal; I pushed him in a wheelchair. Like a housewife, he was in the habit of clipping coupons. Whenever he saw something for sale, he would cut the ad out of the paper and save it for Minna. That made me feel that he must have been a considerate husband willing to share lots of things with his wife. Now, with my help, he enjoyed frequenting the stores in Flushing. For food, he claimed he liked freshwater fish, perch, carp, eel, dace, bullhead, but he wouldn't eat seafood, or anything from the sea except for scallops. The last was recommended by the young nurse because it contained little cholesterol. She also told me to give him milk and cheese, but he disliked them.

One afternoon we went out shopping again. As we were approaching a newsstand on Main Street, Mr. Sheng cried, "Halt!"

"What?" I stopped in my tracks. People were pouring out of the subway exit.

"Wait here," he told me.

"Why?"

"She's coming."

I wanted to ask him more but held back. His mind could hardly take in a regular sentence. If I asked him a question longer than ten words, he wouldn't know how to answer.

More people were passing by, and the two of us stood in the midst of the dwindling crowd. When no passengers were coming out of the exit anymore, I asked him, "Still waiting?"

"Yeah." He rested his hands on his legs. Beside him, a scrap of newspaper was taped to the top horizontal bar of the wheelchair.

"We must buy the fish, remember?" I pointed at the ad.

He looked vacant, his pupils roving from side to side. At this point the subway exit was again swarmed with people, and pedestrians were passing back and forth on the sidewalk. To my amazement, Mr. Sheng lifted his hand at a young lady wearing maroon pants, a pink silk shirt, and wire-rimmed glasses. She hesitated, then stopped. "What can I do for you, Uncle?" she said with a Cantonese accent.

"Seen my wife?" he asked.

"Who's she? What's her name?"

He remained silent and turned his worried face up to me. I stepped in and said, "Her name is Molei Wan." Not knowing how to explain further without offending him, I just winked at the woman.

"I don't know anyone who has that name." She smiled and shook her dark-complected face.

"You're lying!" he yelled.

She glared at him, her nostrils flaring. I pulled her aside and whispered, "Miss, don't take it to heart. He has a mental disorder."

"If he's a sicko, don't let him come out to make others unhappy." She shot me a dirty look and walked away, her shoulder-length hair swaying.

Annoyed, I stepped back to his chair. "Don't speak to a stranger again," I said.

He didn't seem to understand, though he looked displeased, probably because he hadn't caught sight of his wife. I pushed him away while he muttered something I couldn't catch.

The fish store was nearby, and we bought a large whitefish, a two-pounder. It was very fresh, with glossy eyes, full scales, and a firm belly. The young man behind the counter gutted it but left the head on, like I told him. By no means could Mr. Sheng eat the whole thing—I would cook only half of it and save the other half for the next day or later. On our way back, he insisted on holding the fish himself. I had tied the top of the plastic bag, so I didn't intervene when he let it lie flat on his lap. Bloody liquid seeped out and soaked the front of his khaki pants, but I didn't notice it. When we got home, I saw the wet patch and thought he had peed. Then I found that neither of his pant legs was wet. "You meant to create more work for me, eh?" I said. "Why didn't you hold the fish right?"

He looked puzzled. Yet he must have meant to be careless with the fish, peeved that I hadn't let him wait longer outside the subway terminal.

I began undressing him for a shower, which I had planned to do that day anyway. As for his pants soiled by the fish blood, I'd wash them later. There was a washer upstairs on the first floor of the house, where his daughter lived with his two grandchildren and her husband, Harry, a pudgy salesman who traveled a lot and was not home most of the time.

I helped Mr. Sheng into the bathtub. He held on to a walker with its wheels locked while I was washing him. I first lathered him all over and then rinsed him with a nozzle. He enjoyed the shower and cooperated as usual, turning this way and that. He let out happy noises when I sprayed warm water on him. He should he pleased, because few health aides would bathe their patients as carefully as I did. I had once worked in a nursing home, where old people were undressed and strapped to chairs with holes in the seats when we gave them showers. We wheeled them into a machine one by one. Like in an auto bath, water would spurt at them from every direction. When we pulled them out, they'd hiccup and shiver like featherless turkeys. Some of the aides would let those they disliked stay there wet and naked for an hour or two.

After toweling off Mr. Sheng, I helped him on with clean clothes and then combed his gray hair, which was still thick and hadn't lost its sheen. I noticed that his fingernails were quite long, with dirt beneath them, but the company's regulations didn't allow me to clip them, for fear of a lawsuit if they got infected. I told him, "Be a good boy. I'm gonna make you a fish soup."

"Yummy." He clucked, showing two gold-capped teeth.

I couldn't drive, so whenever Mr. Sheng went to see the doctor in the hospital, Minna would take both of us there in her minivan. She already had her hands full with her four-year-old twin boys and her job in a bank, and had to use a babysitter. Her father didn't believe in Western medicine and became unhappy whenever we visited the hospital. He might have his reasons—according to the young nurse who came every other day, acupuncture and medicinal herbs might be more effective in treating his illness. But he would have to pay for the herbs since Medicare didn't cover them. Even so, he'd make me push him from one herbal store to another, and sometimes he went there just to see how those doctors, unlicensed here because of their poor English, treated patients—feeling their pulses, performing cupping, giving therapeutic massages, setting bones. He couldn't afford a whole set of herbs prescribed by a doctor, usually more than a dozen per prescription, but he'd buy something from time to time, a couple of scorpions or centipedes, or a pack of ginseng beard, which is at least ten times cheaper than the roots and which he asked me to steep in piping-hot water to make a tea for him. He would also have me bake and grind the insects and promise him never to disclose his taking them to Minna, who regarded Chinese medicine as quackery. I had no idea if centipedes and scorpions could help him, but whenever he ate a few, he would grow animated for hours, his eyes shedding a tender light while color came to his face. He'd sing folk songs, one after another. He always got the lines garbled, but the melodies were there. Familiar with those songs, I often hummed along with him.

Together we'd sing: "As the limpid brook is babbling east, / I shall keep your words secret and sweet." Or, "A little pouch with a golden string, / Made for me by the village girl / Who smiles like a blooming spring."

But often I wasn't so happy with him. Most of the time he was difficult and grouchy and would throw a tantrum out of the blue. Because Medicare covered acupuncture, he went to a clinic for the treatment regularly. The only acupuncturist within walking distance and listed by the program was Dr. Li, who practiced in one of the tenements on Forty-sixth Avenue. I often missed his office when I took Mr. Sheng there because those brick buildings appeared identical. One afternoon as I was pushing him along the sidewalk shaded by maples with purple leaves, he stopped me, saying we had just passed Dr. Li's clinic. I looked around and figured that he might be correct, so we turned and headed for the right entrance.

Excited about my mistake, he told the doctor I was "a dope." Lying on a sloping bed with needles in his feet, he pointed at his head and said, "My memory's better now."

"Indeed." Dr. Li echoed, "you've improved a lot."

I hated that donkey-faced man, who lied to him. Mr. Sheng couldn't even remember what he'd eaten for lunch. How could anyone in his right mind say his memory had gotten better? He smiled like an idiot, his face showing smugness. I was pretty sure that he had identified the right entrance only by a fluke. Outraged, I flopped down into his wheelchair and pretended to be trembling like him. I groaned, "Oh, help me! Take me to Dr. Li. I need him to stick his magic needles into my neck."

Li laughed, quacking like a duck, while Mr. Sheng fixed his eyes on me like a pair of tiny arrowheads. Red patches were appearing on his cheeks and a tuft of hair suddenly stood up on his crown. That frightened me and I got out of the chair. Even so, I couldn't help but add, "Take me back. I can't walk by myself."

I shouldn't have aped him, speaking out of turn. For the rest of the day he went on jerking his head away from me, even though I cooked his favorite food—chicken porridge with chestnuts in it. I thought he must hate me and would make endless trouble for me. But the next morning he was himself again and even gave me a smile of recognition when I stepped into his quarters in the basement.

Mr. Sheng developed a strange habit—he would prevent me from leaving him alone and want me to sit by him all the time. Even when I went upstairs to launder his clothes, he'd get impatient, making terrible noises. He just needed my attention, I guessed. When I walked out of his room, I could feel his eyes following me. And he had become more obedient at mealtimes and would swallow whatever I fed him. One morning I asked him teasingly, pointing at my nose, "What's my name?"

He managed to say, "Jufen."

I gave him a one-armed hug, thrilled that he'd remembered my name. To be honest, I liked to stay with him, not only because I got paid eight dollars an hour but also because his fondness for me made my work easier. It took less time to feed and bathe him now. He was so happy and mild these days that even his grandchildren would come down to see him. He also went up to visit them when his son-in-law wasn't home. Somehow he seemed afraid of Harry, a white man with thick shoulders, shortish legs, and intense blue eyes. Minna told me that her husband feared that Mr. Sheng might hurt their children and that, besides, Harry didn't like the old man's smell. But honest to God, in my care, my patient didn't stink anymore.

He had quite a number of friends in the neighborhood, and we often went to a small park on Bowne Street to meet them. They were all in their sixties or seventies, three or four women while the other seven or eight were men. But unlike my charge, they weren't ill; they were more clear-headed. Though Mr. Sheng could no longer chat with them, I could see that they used to be quite chummy. They'd tease him good-naturedly, but he never said anything and just smiled at them. One afternoon, Old Peng, a chunky man with a bullet shaped head, asked him loudly, "Who's this? Your girlfriend?" He pointed his thumb at me, its nail ringwormed like a tiny hoof.

To my surprise, Mr. Sheng nodded yes.

"When are you gonna marry her?" a toothless man asked.

"Next month?" a small woman butted in, holding a fistful of pistachios.

Mr. Sheng looked muddled while his friends kept rolling, some waving at me. My face burning, I told them, "Don't make fun of him. Shame on you!"

"She's fierce," said Old Peng.

"Like a little hot pepper," another man echoed.

"She's real good at protecting her man," added the same woman.

I realized there was no way to stop them, so I told Mr. Sheng, "Come, let's go home."

As I was pushing him away, more jesting voices rose behind us. I began to take him to the park less often; instead we'd go to the Flushing Library. He liked to thumb through the magazines there, especially those with photographs.

One morning, as I was scrubbing him in the bathtub, he grasped my hand and pulled it toward him slowly but firmly. I thought he needed me to check a spot bothering him, but to my astonishment, he pressed my hand on his hairy belly, then down to his genitals. Before I could pull it back, he began mumbling. I looked up and saw his eyes giving out a strange light, some sparks flitting in them. Wordlessly I withdrew my hand and went on spraying water on his hack. He kept saying, "I love you, I love you, you know."

Hurriedly I toweled him and helped him into a change of clean clothes. I didn't say a word the whole time, but my mind was in turmoil. How should I handle this? Should I talk to his daughter about this turn of events? He wasn't a bad man, but I didn't love him. Besides our age difference, twenty-one years, I simply couldn't imagine having an intimate relationship with a man again. My ex-husband had left me eight years ago for an old flame of his, a woman entrepreneur in the porcelain business in the Bay Area, and I was accustomed to living alone and never considered remarrying. I'd been treating Mr. Sheng well mainly with an eye to making him like and trust me so my work would be easier, but how should I cope with this madness?

Having no clue what to do, I pretended I didn't understand him. I began to distance myself from him and stay out of his way. Still, I had to take him outdoors and I had to coax him like a child at mealtimes. Also, he'd break into a cry and let loose a flood of tears if I said something harsh to him. He'd murmur my name in a soft voice—"Jufen . . . Jufen . . . ," as if chewing the word. He could have been interesting and charming if he weren't so sick. I felt sorry for him, so I tried to be patient.

About a week later, he began to touch me whenever he could. He'd pat my behind when I stood up to get something for him. He'd also rest his fingers on my forearm as if to prevent me from going away and as if I enjoyed this intimacy. Finally, one afternoon I removed his hand from the top of my thigh and said, "Take your paw off of me. I don't like it."

He was stunned, then burst out wailing. "No fun! No fun!" he cried, pushing the air with his open hand while his face twisted, his eyes shut.

Minna heard the commotion and came down, a huge bun of hair on top of her head. At the sight of her heartbroken father, she asked sharply. "Aunt Niu, what have you done to him?"

"He—he kept harassing me, making advances, so I just told him to stop."

"What? You're a liar. He can hardly know who you are, how could he do anything like that?" Her fleshy face scrunched up, showing that she resolved to defend her father's honor.

"He likes me—that's the truth."

"He's not himself anymore. How could he have normal feelings for you?"

"He said he loved me. Ask him."

She placed her hand, dimpled at the knuckles, on his bony shoulder and shook him. "Dad, tell me, do you love Jufen?"

He looked at her blankly, as if in confusion. I hated him for keeping mute and humiliating me like this.

Minna straightened up and said to me, "Obviously you are lying. You hurt him, but you pinned the blame on him."

"Damn it, I told you the truth!"

"How can you prove that?"

"If you don't believe me, all right, I quit." I was surprised by what I said; this job was precious to me, but it was too late to retract my words.

She smirked, fluttering her mascaraed eyelashes. "Who are you? You think you're so indispensable that the Earth will stop spinning without you?"

Speechless, I walked into the doorway to collect my things. It was late afternoon, almost time to call it a day. I knew Minna had befriended Ning Zhang, the owner of my agency; they both came from Nanjing. The bitch would definitely bad-mouth me to that man to make it hard for me to land another job. Even so, I had to keep up appearances and would never beg her to take me back.

I didn't eat dinner, and I wept for hours that night. Yet I didn't regret having given Minna a piece of my mind. As I anticipated, my boss, Ning Zhang, called early the next morning and told me not to go to work anymore.

For several days I stayed home watching TV. I liked Korean and Taiwanese shows, but I wanted to learn some English, so I watched soaps, *All My Children* and *General Hospital*, which I could hardly understand. Using a friend as an interpreter, I talked to Father Lorenzo of our church about my job loss; he said I shouldn't lose heart. "God will provide, and you'll find work soon," he assured me. "At the moment you should use the free time to attend an English class here."

I didn't reply and thought, Easier said than done. At my age, how can I learn another language from scratch? I couldn't even remember the order of the alphabet. If only I were thirty years younger!

Then one evening Ning Zhang called, saying he'd like to have me take care of Mr. Sheng again. Why? I wondered to myself. Didn't they send over another health aide? I asked him, "What happened? Minna's not angry with me anymore?"

"No. She just has a short temper, you know that. Truth be told, since you left, her dad often refuses to eat, sulking like a child, so we want you to go back."

"What makes you think I'll do that?"

"I know you. You're kindhearted and will never see an old man suffer and starve because of your self-pride."

That was true, so I agreed to restart the next morning. Ning Zhang thanked me and said he'd give me a raise at the end of the year.

Minna was quite friendly when I returned to work. Her father resumed eating normally, though he still wouldn't stop saying he loved me and he would touch me whenever he could. I didn't reproach him—I just avoided body contact so I might not hurt his feelings again. To be fair, he was obsessed but innocuous. It was the incurable illness that had reduced him to such a wreck; otherwise, some older woman might have married him willingly. Whenever we ran into a friend of his on the street or in the library, Mr. Sheng would say I was his girlfriend. I was embarrassed but didn't bother to correct him. There're things that the more you try to explain, the more complicated they become. I kept mum, telling myself I was only doing my job.

Once in a while he would get assertive, attempting to make me touch his genitals when I bathed him, or trying to fondle my breasts. He even began calling me "my old woman." Irritated, I griped to Minna in private, "We have to find a way to stop him or I can't continue to work like this."

"Aunt Niu," she sighed, "let us be honest with each other. I'm terribly worried too. Tell me, do you have feelings for my dad?"

"What do you mean?" I was puzzled.

"I mean, do you love him?"

"No, I don't."

She gave me a faint smile as if to say no woman would openly admit her affection for a man. I wanted to stress that at most I might like him a little, but she spoke before I could. "How about marrying him? I mean just in appearance."

"What a silly thing to say. How could I support myself if I don't hold a job?"

"That's why I said just in appearance."

I was more baffled. "I don't get it."

"I mean, you can keep your job but live in this apartment, pretending to be his wife. Just to make him content and peaceful. I'll pay you four hundred dollars a month. Besides, you'll keep your wages."

"Well, I'm not sure." I couldn't see what she was really driving at.

She pressed on. "It will work like this—legally you're not his spouse at all. Nothing will change except that you'll spend more time with him in here."

"I don't have to share his bed?"

"Absolutely not. You can set up your own quarters in there." She pointed at the storage room, which was poky but could be turned into a cozy nest.

"So the marriage will be just in name?"

"Exactly."

"Let me think about it, okay?"

"Sure, no need to rush."

It took me two days to decide to accept the offer. I had remembered my aunt, who in her early forties had married a paraplegic nineteen years older and nursed him to his grave. She wasn't even fond of the man but took pity on him. In a way, she sacrificed herself so that her family wouldn't starve. When her husband died, she didn't inherit anything from him—he left his house to his nephew. Later she went to join her daughter from her first marriage and is still staying with my cousin in a small town on the Yellow River. Compared with my aunt, I was in a much better position, earning wages for myself. Eventually if I moved into Mr. Sheng's place, I might not have to rent my apartment anymore and plus could save eighty-one dollars a month on the subway pass. When I told Minna of my acceptance, she was delighted and said I was kindness itself.

To my surprise, she came again in the afternoon with a sheet of paper and asked me to sign it, saying this was just a statement of the terms we'd agreed on. I couldn't read English, so I wanted to see a Chinese version. I had to be careful about signing anything; four years ago I'd lost my deposit when I left Elmhurst for Corona to share an apartment with a friend—my former landlord wouldn't refund me the seven hundred dollars and showed me the cosigned agreement that stated I would give up the money if I moved out before the lease expired.

Minna said she'd rewrite the thing in Chinese. The next morning, as I was seated beside Mr. Sheng and reading a newspaper article to him, Minna stepped in and motioned for me to come into the kitchen. I went over, and she handed me the agreement. I read through it and felt outraged. It sounded like I was planning to swindle her father out of his property. The last paragraph stated: "To sum up, Jufen Niu agrees that she shall never enter into matrimony with Jinping Sheng or accept any inheritance from him. Their 'union' shall remain nominal forever."

I asked Minna, "So you think I'm a gold digger, huh? If you don't trust me, why bother about this fake marriage in the first place?"

"I do trust you, Aunt Niu, but we're in America now, where even the air can make people change. We'd better spell out everything on paper before-hand. To tell the truth, my dad owns two apartments, which he bought many years ago when real estate was cheap in this area, so we ought to pre-vent any trouble down the road."

"I never thought he was rich, but I won't 'marry' him, period."

She fixed her cat eyes on me and said, "Then how can you continue work-ing here?"

"I won't."

"I didn't mean to offend you, Aunt Niu. Can't we leave this open and talk about it later when we both calm down?"

"I just don't feel I can sell myself this way. I don't love him. You know how hard it is for a woman to marry a man she doesn't love."

She smirked. I knew what she was thinking—for a woman my age, it was foolish to take love into account when offered a marriage. Indeed, love gets scarcer as we grow older. All the same, I nerved myself and said, "This is my last day."

"Well, maybe not." She turned and made for the door, her hips jiggling a little. She shouldn't have worn jeans, which made her appear more rotund.

Ning Zhang called the next day and asked me to come to his office down-town for "a heart-to-heart talk." I told him I wouldn't feel comfortable con-fiding anything to a thirtysomething like him. In fact, he was pushing forty and already looked middle-aged, stout in the midriff and with a shiny bald spot like a lake in the mouth of an extinct volcano. Still, he insisted that I come over, so I agreed to see him the next morning.

For a whole day I thought about what to say to him. Should I refuse to look after Mr. Sheng no matter what? I wasn't sure, because I was in Ning Zhang's clutches. He could keep me out of work for months or even for years. Should I sign the humiliating agreement with Minna? Perhaps I had no choice but to accept it. How about asking for a raise? That might be the only possible gain I could get. So I decided to bargain with my boss for a one-dollar-an-hour raise.

Before setting out the next morning, I combed my hair, which was mostly black, and I also made up my face a little. I was amazed to see myself in the mirror: jutting cheekbones, bright eyes, and a water-chestnut-shaped mouth. If twenty years younger, I could have been a looker. Better yet, I still had a small waistline and a bulging chest. I left home, determined to confront my boss.

At the subway station I chanced on a little scarecrow of a woman who pulled a baby carriage loaded with sacks of plastic bottles and aluminum cans. No doubt she was Chinese and over seventy, in brown slacks and a black short-sleeved shirt printed with yellow hibiscuses. The cloth sacks holding the containers were clean and colored like pieces of baggage. A rusty folding stool was bound to the top of the huge load. On the side of the tiny buggy hung a string pouch holding a bottle of water and a little blue bag with a red tassel, obviously containing her lunch. There were also three large sacks, trussed together, separated from the buggy-load, and holding two liter Coke bottles. All the people on the platform kept a distance from this white-haired woman. She looked neat and gentle but restless, and went on tightening the ropes wrapped around the load. A fiftyish man passed by with two little girls sporting loopy honey-colored curls, and the kids turned to gawk at the sacks of containers and at the old woman, who waved her small hand and said to them with a timid smile, "Bye-bye." Neither of the wide-eyed girls responded.

The train came and discharged passengers. I helped the crone pull her stuff into the car. She was so desperate to get her things aboard that she didn't even thank me after the door slid shut. She was panting hard. How many bottles and cans has she here? I wondered. Probably about two hundred. She stood by the door, afraid she wouldn't be able to get all her stuff off at her destination. Time and again I glanced at her, though no one else seemed to notice her at all. She must have been a daily passenger with a similar load.

A miserable feeling was welling in me. In that withered woman I saw myself. How many years could I continue working as a health aide who was never paid overtime or provided with any medical insurance or a retirement plan? Would I ever make enough to lay aside some for my old age? How would I support myself when I could no longer attend to patients? I must do something now, or I might end up like that little crone someday, scavenging through garbage for cans and bottles to sell to a recycling shop. The more I thought about her, the more despondent I became.

The woman got off at Junction Boulevard, dragging away her load that was five times larger than her body. People hurried past her, and I was afraid she might fall at the stairs if one of her sacks snagged on something.

Her flimsy sneakers seemed to be held together by threads as she shuffled away, pulling the baby carriage while the three huge sacks on her back quivered.

Ning Zhang was pleased to see me when I stepped into his office. "Take a seat, Jufen," he said. "Anything to drink?"

"No." I shook my head and sat down before his desk.

"Tell me, how can I persuade you to go back to Minna's?"

"I want a pension plan!" I said firmly.

He was taken aback, then grinned. "Are you kidding me? You know our agency doesn't offer that and can't set a precedent."

"I know. That's why I won't go look after Mr. Sheng anymore."

"But he might die soon if he continues refusing to eat."

Pity suddenly gripped my heart, but I got hold of myself. I said, "He'll get over it, he'll be fine. He doesn't really know me that well. Besides, he has a memory like a bucket riddled with holes."

"Do you understand, if you don't work for us, you may not be able to work elsewhere either?"

"I've made up my mind that from now on I'll work only for a company that provides a pension plan."

"That means you'll have to be able to speak English"

"I can learn."

"At your age? Give me a break. How many years have you been in this country? Ten or eleven? How many English sentences can you speak? Five or six?"

"From now on I'll live differently. If I can't speak enough English to work for a unionized company, I'll starve and die!"

The determination in my voice must have impressed him. He breathed a sigh and said, "Quite frankly, I admire that, that jolt of spirit, although you make me feel like a capitalist exploiter. All right, I wish you the best of luck. If I can do anything for you, let me know."

When I came out of his office, the air pulsed with the wings of seagulls and was full of the aroma of kebabs. The trees were green and sparkling with dewdrops in the sunshine. My head was a little light with the emotion still surging in my chest. To be honest, I'm not sure if I'll be able to learn enough English to live a different life, but I must try.

33

A Bad Day for Pisces

✺ *Fran Pokras Yariv*

I believe in signs and in the stars, and it must have been a bad day for Pisces the day Ms. Breur-Gordon called me, Ofelia Hernandez wrote in her journal, the one her friend Corrine gave her for her birthday, *so I should've said no when she asked me to work for her mother, but I needed the money.*

Ofelia put the pen down and took a sip of her Coke. She was sitting in the employee lounge of Sunset Hills Retirement Community while little Mrs. Breur was in the living room with the other residents watching the entertainment and snacking on wine and cheese. Ofelia could hear the singer even though the door to the lounge was closed. He came every three weeks and sang the same old songs, and all the residents seemed to know the words. She looked at her watch. She still had a good half hour before she'd have to go get Mrs. Breur and take her up to her room for a rest.

Ofelia reread the sentence she'd just written. It was true she did need the money if she was ever going to move out and get her own place because if she stayed at home any longer she'd really go crazy and anyway, she wasn't getting any younger.

Almost thirty! How did *that* happen!!! When she was in high school, she was sure that by the time she was twenty-six she'd be married with a couple of kids, but that wasn't the way it turned out. But better than Corrine, who'd gotten knocked up senior year and had three kids and was living with her husband in his parents' house. She wouldn't change places with Corrine for anything.

Ofelia turned the page in her journal and drew a long line down the middle to make two columns. At the top of the first column she printed the heading *Good Things about Working for Mrs. Breur.* On the other side she printed *Bad Things about Working for Mrs. Breur.* This was something her father had taught her to do. Ofelia wondered, not for the first time, if he'd made a list like that before he ran off with that slut, Ana.

Fran Pokras Yariv, "A Bad Day for Pisces," from *Feeding Mrs. Moskovitz and The Caregiver,* by Barbara Pokras and Fran Pokras Yariv, 2010. Reprinted by permission of Syracuse University Press and the author.

In the Good Things column, she wrote *1. Pay is good.* Underneath she carefully listed the other positives. *2. I get paid on time. 3. Mrs. Breur is nice.* She wrote the number 4, but she couldn't think of anything else. How pathetic was that! So she began on the Bad Things side. That was easier. *1. Ms. Breur-Gordon. 2. Ms. Breur-Gordon. 3. Ms. Breur-Gordon.* She listed the numbers 4 through 10 and made ditto marks down the page. Ms. Breur-Gordon!

Even though Ms. Breur-Gordon had a big-deal job at an ad agency, the only thing she seemed to care about was her little old mother. She was always snooping around to make sure everybody was treating her right. One of the aides—Buddies was what they were called at Sunset Hills—warned Ofelia when she started the job that she was the fourth caregiver Ms. Breur-Gordon had hired that year. She had fired one of them and two had quit. No wonder the Buddies, the nurse, even Janice, the director, were all scared of her.

When she'd said okay to Ms. Breur-Gordon, Ofelia had been sure she could handle it. She'd been a full time aide at Pacific Villa in Santa Monica for a year and a half and had put up with all the politics. Aides were always quitting or getting fired, which meant the ones who hung in worked like donkeys. But when corporate fired the director and brought in that witch, Karla, Ofelia had had enough.

After Pacific Villa she worked for an agency, which meant that they sent her out on jobs for anywhere from a few hours to a few weeks, and she never knew what she'd get. It's not like I asked for so much, Ofelia thought, just a steady job with nice people and decent pay. She didn't understand why that was so hard. Anyway, she was really sick and tired of the agency, so when Ms. Breur-Gordon called, Ofelia was ready to take on a full-time private job.

Old Mrs. Breur wasn't in such bad shape compared to some of the others, Ofelia thought when she first met her. She was a skinny little thing, all bent over, and used a walker but she could go to the toilet herself. She wouldn't have to be changing diapers. Not yet, at least. Ofelia knew her official job would be helping her get dressed, doing her laundry, and walking her down to the dining room and to the activities. That was all she was really required to do, but Ms. Breur-Gordon made it clear that she expected much more.

"I don't want poor Mother just sitting in her room," Ms. Breur-Gordon had told Ofelia when she started the job. "I want her to have friends and to have an active lifestyle."

Well, yeah, Ofelia thought. That would be nice except that little Mrs. Breur was hard of hearing and didn't talk much and she didn't like any of the activities except bingo and nobody talked when they played bingo.

Bingo was serious business because the winner got these coupons called Sunset Bucks they could use to buy things like shampoo and candy. And sometimes little Mrs. Breur just wanted to take a nap instead of going downstairs to hear a lecture on diabetes or watch a movie. What did Ms. Breur-Gordon want her to do, Ofelia wondered, drag her mother out of bed and force her to go downstairs? But if Ms. Breur-Gordon called and her mother was in her room instead of taking part in an activity, she had a fit. And she would say to Ofelia in that voice Ofelia had come to dread, "Now, Ofelia, you know I expect Mother to socialize."

No wonder Ofelia was always nervous just knowing that Ms. Breur-Gordon could show up out of nowhere and inspect the apartment and ask questions like did Mother eat all her lunch, what did she eat, did you wash her hair, were the sheets changed, and on and on. Once Ofelia forgot to sign Mrs. Breur up for an outing to the museum and you would've thought she'd poisoned her the way Ms. Breur-Gordon carried on. Ofelia felt like telling her if you're so concerned, why don't you take her to live in your big house and care for her yourself, like we do in my culture. But of course she kept her mouth shut. But Ms. Breur-Gordon must have felt bad because the next day she brought Ofelia a big box of chocolates. After that, when the weekly activity schedule came out, Ofelia made sure she was the first one down at the desk to sign Mrs. Breur up.

Money isn't everything, Ofelia wrote at the bottom of the page with the columns. Just because you were rich didn't mean you were happy or were a good person. All she had to do was look around Sunset Hills to figure that out. They didn't take any Medi-Cal people, and they charged big bucks, and on top of that they kept raising the rent and the cost of all the extras like daily housekeeping and personal laundry. She figured that the residents were rich or had rich children like Ms. Breur-Gordon, but not too many of the old people, except maybe those with Alzheimer's, looked happy. Mrs. Breur sure didn't look happy, even when she had her hair and her nails done. But then again, Ofelia knew that being poor didn't make a person happy either. Her mother was proof of that. She was a server in the cafeteria at Harding Junior High, and the little money they paid her she ended up giving to Ofelia's spoiled brother, who couldn't keep a job. She was always sighing and complaining, so you couldn't call her happy.

But if I had a choice I'd rather have money because then I wouldn't have to always worry that Ms. Breur-Gordon was going to fire me, Ofelia wrote.

The door opened and Connie came in balancing a small tray with a plate of fruit and cheese and a glass of wine in one hand. The Buddies weren't supposed to drink at the wine and cheese hours, but nobody except the Filipinas paid any attention to that rule.

Ofelia closed her journal. Connie was her favorite Buddy because she was friendly, and, besides, she always had all the latest gossip, which was why Ofelia wouldn't let her read anything she wrote in her journal.

Connie put the tray on the table and sat down across from Ofelia. "Want some cheese?" She pushed the plate toward her.

"Thanks." Ofelia took a little square of cheddar and a cracker.

"It is too funny out there." Connie grinned. "Mr. Grant is guzzling that cheap wine like he was in a desert and it was water! And him with diabetes!"

Ofelia giggled. Mr. Grant was a character, all right. He was always cracking dirty jokes and flirting, even worse sometimes grabbing at any female who was dumb enough to get near him. When she first started working at Sunset Hills, Mr. Grant pinched her butt when she walked by his table in the dining room. Anybody else and Ofelia would've told him off, but Mr. Grant was just like that and didn't really mean anything, so she just said, "Hey, Mr. Grant, you're way too old for me," and he said something like "but I'm young at heart." So Ofelia just laughed and said, "Well, you have to show me your portfolio before you can touch me!" and everybody at his table laughed.

Ofelia heard applause from the living room. Connie rolled her eyes, gulped down her wine, and popped a couple of pieces of cheese in her mouth. Break time was over.

People were still in the living room even though most of the food was gone. The singer was talking to Mr. Grosso, who used to play the piano for one of those big bands, and a couple of the women who had crushes on Mr. Grosso were hanging around. Mrs. Breur was sitting on the couch next to Gerri Kane, and she seemed to be having a good time, so Ofelia decided to have some cheese and crackers.

She stood in back of Debby, the activities director, and Emma Greenberg who was helping herself to some cheese from the platter.

"How about a glass of wine, Mrs. Greenberg," Debby asked in that fake cheery voice.

"No, thanks," Mrs. Greenberg said loudly. "When you spring for some decent wine, maybe I'll indulge."

Debby turned all red, and Ofelia tried not to laugh. Mrs. Greenberg always said what was on her mind, and she didn't care who heard. A couple of women gave Ms. Greenberg dirty looks, but Mr. Grant, who was standing nearby, gave one of his loud "ha-ha" laughs.

"Right on, Emma!" he said. "This stuff's rotgut. Must've got it at the 99-Cent Store."

Debby turned away from them and walked toward the piano, where the singer and Mr. Grosso were still talking. Emma made a face at her back, and Mr. Grant laughed again. Ofelia knew that was why a lot of the residents were afraid of Mr. Grant and Mrs. Greenberg—you never knew what they'd say next. But Ofelia kind of admired them. Not many people, herself included, said what they really thought. Especially not at Sunset Hills.

It was a good thing that Ms. Greenberg didn't need a full time caregiver, Ofelia thought, because with her mouth, she'd really be a handful. She put a square of cheese on a cracker and sighed. Maybe working for little Mrs. Breur wasn't so bad after all.

34

Wheelchair

&*Lewis Nordan*

Winston Krepps had been abandoned by his attendant, and the door was shut tight.

Winston pressed the control lever of his chair. The battery was low, so the motor sounded strained. The chair turned in a slow circular motion; the rubber tires squeaked on the linoleum floor of the kitchen.

For a moment, as the chair turned, Winston saw two teenaged boys on a bridge. Winston released the control lever, and the chair stopped. The boys were naked and laughing, and the Arkansas sky was bright blue. Winston recognized himself as one of the two boys. He pushed the hallucination away from his eyes. It was the day real life had ended, he thought.

The clock above the refrigerator said four—that would be Thursday. Harris, his attendant, must have left on Monday.

Winston turned his chair again and faced the living room. He saw a boy lying on his back on a white table. Winston turned his head and tried not to see. Doctors and nurses moved through the room. The prettiest of the nurses stood by the table and chatted with the boy. The boy—it was Winston, he could not prevent recognizing himself—was embarrassed at his nakedness, but he could not move to cover himself. An X-ray machine was rolled into place. The pretty nurse said, "Don't breathe now." The boy thought he might ask her out when he was better, if she wasn't too old for him. He had not understood yet that this was the day sex ended. Winston looked away and pressed the lever of the chair.

The motor hummed and he rolled toward the bedroom. The tires squeaked on the linoleum, then were silent on the carpet. The motor strained to get through the carpet, but it did not stop. Monday, then, was the last day he was medicated.

Winston negotiated the little S-curve in the hallway. He could see into

Lewis Nordan, "Wheelchair," from *Welcome to the Arrow-Catcher Fair: Stories.* (Baton Rouge: Louisiana State University Press, 1983). Later in *Sugar Among the Freaks: Selected Stories* (Front Porch, 1996). Originally in *Arkansas Times Magazine.* Copyright © 1983 *Arkansas Times.* Reprinted by permission.

the bathroom. The extra leg-bag was draped over the edge of the tub, the detergents and irrigation fluids and medications were lined up on the cabinet. Winston saw his mother in the bathroom, but as if she were still young and were standing in the kitchen of her home. He saw himself near her, still a boy, strapped into his first wheelchair.

He closed his eyes, but he could still see. His mother was washing dewberries in the sink. There were clean pint mason jars on the cabinet and a large blue enamel cooker on the stove. His mother said, "The stains! I don't know if dewberries are worth the trouble." Winston watched, against his will, the deliberateness of her cheer, the artificiality of it.

He stopped his chair in the bedroom. There was the table Harris had built, the attendant who had abandoned him. Harris had been like a child the night he finished the table, he was so proud of himself. He even skipped that night at the countrywestern disco, where he spent most of his time, just to sit home with Winston and have the two of them admire it together. Winston resented the table now, and the feelings he had had, briefly, for Harris. How could a person build you a table and sit with you that night and look at it, and then leave you alone. It was easy to hate Harris.

He looked at the articles that made up the contents of the room—his typewriter, his lamp, and books and papers, a poem he had been trying to write, still in the typewriter. His typing stick was on the floor, where he had dropped it by accident on Monday.

Then Harris stepped into the line of Winston's vision. Winston had not realized you could hallucinate forward as well as back, but he was not surprised. It was the same worthless Harris. "I'm a boogie person, man," Harris seemed to explain. He was wearing tight jeans and no shirt, his feet were bare. He was tall and slender and straight. "I'm into boogie, it's into me." Winston said, "But you built me a table, Harris." Then he said nothing at all.

Winston's hunger had stopped some time ago, he couldn't remember just when. He knew his face was flushed from lack of medication. His leg-bag had been full for a couple of days, so urine seeped out of the stoma for a while. It had stopped now that he was dehydrated.

Winston heard cars passing on the paved road outside his window. He had cried out until his voice was gone. He imagined bright Arkansas skies and a sweet-rank fragrance of alfalfa hay and manure and red clover on the wind from the pastures outside town. He thought of telephone wires singing in the heat.

Winston looked back at the floor again, at his typing stick. The stick made him remember Monday, the day Harris left, and before Winston knew he was abandoned.

He had been in his chair at the kitchen table with his plastic drinking straw in his mouth. He was sipping at the last of a pitcher of water. The time alone had been pleasant for him—none of Harris's music playing, none of his TV game shows or ridiculous friends and their conversation about cowboy disco and girls and the rest. Winston sipped on the water and felt the top of the plastic tube with his tongue.

He pressed his tongue over the hole in the tube and felt the circle it made there. He thought he could have counted all the taste buds enclosed within the circle if he tried. He thought of his father holding a duck call to his lips to show Winston how to hold his tongue when he was a child, before the accident. Winston remembered taking the call from his father's hand, and he wondered if that touching were not the last touch of love he had felt—the last in the real world anyway, and so the last. The touching of the tube to his tongue brought his father back to him, the smell of alligator grass in the winter swamp, a fragrance of fresh tobacco and wool and shaving lotion and rubber hip waders, and more that he had forgotten from that world.

He had gone to his typewriter and had meant to write what he remembered. He had almost been able to believe it would restore him, undo what was done.

He had rolled up to the table, as close as the chair would take him. The stick with the rubber tips was lying on the table with four or five inches sticking out over the edge. Winston used his single remaining shoulder muscle to push his left hand forward onto the table. His fingers had long ago stiffened into a permanent curl. He maneuvered the hand until the typing stick was between his second and third fingers.

At last he dragged it close enough to his face. He clenched one end of the stick between his teeth and tasted the familiar rubber grip. He steadied himself and aimed the stick at the *on* button of his typewriter. The machine buzzed and clacked and demanded attention. For an instant, as he always did when he heard this sound, he felt genuinely alive, an inhabitant of a real world, a real life. And not just life—it was power he felt, almost that. Writing—just for a moment, but always for that moment—was real. It was dancing. It was getting the girl and the money and kicking sand in the face of the bully. He began, letter by letter, to type with the stick in his mouth.

When he had finished, what he had written was not good. The words he saw on the page were not what he had meant. What he had felt seemed trivial now, and hackneyed. He said, "Shit." He touched the *off* button and shut the typewriter down.

He tried to drop the stick from his mouth onto x the table again, but the effort of writing had exhausted him. The stick hit the table, but it had been dropped hastily, impatiently, and it did not fall where Winston had intended. It rolled onto his lap, across his right leg, where he could not reach it. Finally it rolled off his leg and onto the floor.

That was on Monday. He could have used the stick now to dial the telephone.

There was a series of three muscle spasms. The first one was mild. Winston's left leg began to rise up toward his face. The spasm continued upward through his body and into his shoulders. For a moment he could not breathe, but then the contraction ended and it was over. His foot settled back into place. He caught his breath again.

When the second spasm began he saw the center of hell. A great bird, encased in ice, flapped its enormous wings and set off storms throughout all its icy regions. In the storms and in the ice was a chant, and the words of the chant were *Ice ice up to the neck.*

Winston's legs, both of them this time, rose up toward his face and hung there for an eternity of seconds. He watched the ice-imprisoned bird and listened to the chant. His legs flailed right and left in the chair. Now they settled down. They jerked out and kicked and crossed one another and flailed sidewise again. Winston's feet did not touch the footrests, and his legs were askew. His shoulders rose up to his ears and caused him to scrunch up the features of his face and to hold his breath against his will.

Then it ended. He could breathe again. It was easy to hate his useless legs and his useless arms and his useless genitals and his insides over which he had no control. He was tilted in his chair, listing twenty degrees to the right.

Winston felt an odd peacefulness settle upon him. He saw a swimming pool and a pavilion in summertime. The bathhouse was green-painted, and the roof was corrugated aluminum. He saw himself at sixteen, almost seventeen. For the first time he did not avert his eyes. A radio was playing, there was a screech of young children on a slide. The boy he watched stood at the pool's edge, a country boy at a town pool, as happy as if he had just begun to live his life inside a technicolor movie.

There was a girl too, a city girl. She told him she was from Memphis, her name was Twilah. There was a blaze of chlorine and Arkansas sun in her hair and eyes. No one could have been more beautiful. Her hair was flaming orange, and a billion freckles covered her face and shoulders and breasts, even her lips and ears. The radio played and the sun shone and the younger children screeched on the slide.

Outside his window, where he could not see it, a bird made a sound—a noise, really—an odd two-noted song, and the song caused the memory to grow more vivid, more heartbreaking. He wanted to see all the places Twilah might hide her freckles. He wanted to count them, to see her armpits and beneath her fingernails and under her clothing. He wanted to examine her tongue and her nipples and forbidden places he could scarcely imagine. It was easy to fall in love when you were sixteen, almost seventeen, and a lifeguard was blowing a steel whistle at a swimmer trespassing beneath a diving board.

※

The third spasm was a large one. It seemed to originate somewhere deep in his body, near the core. The tingle in his face that signaled it was like a jangle of frantic bells rung in warning.

He imagined great flocks of seabirds darkening the air above an island. He saw wildlife scurrying for shelter.

Motion had begun in his body now. His legs were rising as if they were lighter than air. Then, suddenly, and for no reason—it may have been merely the nearness of death—Winston did not care what his legs did. He watched them in bemusement. For the first time since the accident, they were not monstrous to him, they were not dwarfish or grotesque. They were his legs, only that. For the first time in seventeen years, he could not discover—or even think to seek—the measure of himself, or of the universe, in his limbs. He was in the grip of a spasm more violent than anything he had ever imagined, in which, for a full minute he could not breathe at all, could not draw breath, and yet he felt as refreshed as if he were breathing sea air a thousand miles from any coast.

He began to see as he had never seen before. He saw as if his seeing were accompanied by an eternal music, as if the past were being presented to him through the vision of an immortal eye. He was not dead—there was no question of that. He was alive, for a little longer anyway, and he was seeing in the knowledge that there is greater doom in not looking than in looking. He fixed his eye—this magical, immortal eye—on a swamp-lake in eastern Arkansas.

In the swamp he saw a cove, and in the cove an ancient tangle of briers and cypress knees and gum stumps. He saw water that was pure but blacker than slate, made mirrorlike by the tannic acid from the cypress trees, and he saw the trees and skies and clouds reflected in its surface.

The eye penetrated the reflecting surface and saw beneath the water. He saw a swamp floor of mud and silt. He saw a billion strings of vegetation and tiny root systems. He saw fish—bright bluegills and silvery crappie, long-snouted gar, and lead-bellied cat with ropy whiskers. He saw turtles and mussels and the earth of plantations sifted there from other states, another age, through a million ditches and on the feet of turkey vultures and blue herons and kingfishers. He saw schools of minnows and a trace of slave death from a century before. He saw baptizings and drownings. He saw the transparent wings of snake doctors, he saw lost fish stringers and submerged logs and the ghosts of lovers.

He saw the boat.

The boat was beneath the surface with the rest, old and colorless and waterlogged. It was not on the bottom, only half-sunk, two feet beneath the surface of the swamp.

The boat was tangled in vegetation, in brambles and briers and the submerged tops of fallen tupelo gums and willows. It was tangled in trotlines and rusted hooks and a faded Lucky 13 and the bale of a minnow bucket and the shreds of a shirt some child took off on a hot day and didn't get home with.

The world that Winston looked into seemed affected by the spasm that he continued to suffer and entertain. Brine flowed into freshets, ditches gurgled with strange water. The willows moved, the trotlines swayed, the crappie did not bite a hook. Limbs of fallen trees shivered under the water, muscadine vines, the sleeve of a boy's shirt waved as if to say good-bye. The gar felt the movement with its long snout, the cat with its ropy whiskers, the baptized child felt it, and the drowned man. The invisible movement of the water stirred the silt and put grit in the mussel's shell. The lost bass plug raised up a single hook as if in question.

And the spasm touched the half-sunken boat.

Winston was breathing again, with difficulty. He was askew in his chair, scarcely sitting at all. He thought his right leg had been broken in the thrashing, but he couldn't tell. He wasn't really interested. He knew he would see what he had been denied—what he had denied himself.

He watched the boat beneath the surface. The boat trembled in the slow, small movement of the waters. The trembling was so slight that it could be seen only by magic, with an eye that could watch for years in the space of this second. Winston watched all the years go past, and all their seasons. Winter summer spring fall. The boat trembled, a brier broke. Oxidation and sedimentation and chance and drought and rain, a crumbling somewhere, a falling away of matter from matter. In the slowness the boat broke free of its constraints.

It rose up closer to the surface and floated twelve inches beneath the tannic mirror of the lake.

The boat could move freely now. Winston was slouched in his chair, crazed with fever but still alive. He knew what he was watching, and he would watch it to the end.

Harris said, "I didn't know you would *die*, man. I never knew boogie could kill anybody." It was tempting to watch Harris, to taunt him for his ignorance, his impossible shallowness, but Winston kept his eye on the boat.

The boat moved through the water. It didn't matter how it moved, by nature or magic or the ripples sent out by a metaphorical storm, it moved beneath the water of a swamp-lake in eastern Arkansas.

It moved past cypress and gum, past a grove of walnut and pecan. It moved past a cross that once was burned on the Winter Quarters side of the lake, it moved past Mrs. Hightower's lake bank where the Methodists held the annual picnic, past the spot where a one-man band made music a long time ago and caused the children to dance, it moved past a brown-and-white cow drinking knee-deep in the Ebeneezer Church's baptizing pool. It moved past Harper's woods and a sunken car and a washed away boat dock. It moved past the Indian mound and past some flooded chicken houses, it moved past the shack where Mr. Long shot himself, it moved past the Kingfisher Café.

And then it stopped. Still twelve inches beneath the water, the boat stopped its movement and rested against the pilings of a narrow bridge above the lake. On the bridge Winston could see two boys—himself one of them—naked and laughing in the sun. Winston did not avert his eyes.

The boys' clothes were piled beside them in a heap. One of the boys—himself, as Winston knew it would be—left the railing of the bridge.

It was part fall, part dive—a fall he would make the most of. It lasted, it seemed, forever. Slow-arching and naked, spraddle-legged, self-conscious, comic, bare-assed, country-boy dive.

There was no way for him to miss the boat, of course. He hit it. The other boy, the terrified child on the bridge, climbed down from the railing and held his clothes to his bare chest and did not jump.

He only had to see it once.

And yet it was not quite over.

Winston's life was being saved, like cavalry arriving in the nick of time. This was not an hallucination, this was real. There was an ambulance team in the little apartment, two men in white uniforms. It was hard to believe, but Harris was there as well—Harris the boogieman, repentant and re-turned, still explaining himself, just as he had in the hallucinations. "Boo-gie is my *life*," he said, as the ambulance team began their work.

Then it began to happen again, the opening of the magical eye. It was focused on Harris. Through it he saw, as he always saw, even with-out magic, the bright exterior of Harris's physical beauty—his slenderness and sexuality and strength and straight back and perfect limbs, and also, somehow, beyond his beauty, which before this moment had been always a perverse mirror in which to view only his, Winston's, own deformity and celibacy and loss, beyond the mirror of his physical perfection and, with clear vision, even in this real but dreamlike room, filled with a hellish blue-flashing light from outside, and with I.V. bottles and injections and an inflatable splint for his leg and the white of sheets and uniforms and the presence also of the apartment manager who had come, a large oily man named Sooey Leonard, he saw past Harris's beauty to the frightened, disorganized, hopeless boy that Harris was. Winston understood, at last, the pain in what Harris told him. Boogie is my life. It was not a thing to be mocked, as Winston had so recently thought. It was not a lame excuse for failure. What was terrifying and painful was that Harris knew exactly what he was saying, and that he meant, in despair, exactly what he said. It was acknowledgment and confession, not excuse, a central failure of intellect and spirit that Harris understood in himself, was cursed to know, and to know also that he could not change, a doom he had carried with him since his conception and could look at, as if it belonged to someone else. The knowledge that Harris knew himself so well and, in despair of it, could prophesy his future, with all its meanness and shallowness and absence of hope, swept through Winston like a wind of grief. He wanted to tell Harris that it wasn't true, that he was not doomed, no matter the magnitude of the failure here. He wanted to remind him of the table he had built and of how they felt together that night it was finished, when they had sat at home alone together and not turned on the television but only sat and looked at the table and talked about it and then made small talk about other things, both of them knowing they were talking about the table. He wanted Harris to know that the table proved him wrong.

He could say nothing. The ambulance team bumped and jolted him onto a stretcher-table and held the clanking I.V. bottles above him.

The sunlight was momentarily blinding as he was wheeled out the door of the apartment and onto the sidewalk. For a moment Winston could see nothing at all, only a kaleidoscope of colors and shapes behind his eyelids.

And yet in the kaleidoscope, by magic he supposed, he found that he could see Harris and himself. They stood—somehow Winston could stand—in the landscape of another planet, with red trees and red rivers and red houses and red farm animals, and through all the atmosphere, as if in a red whirlwind, flew the small things of Winston's life: the typewriter and the failed poem in it, the battery charger for his chair, and the water mattress and the sheepskin, the chair itself and the leather strap that held him in it, his spork—the combination spoon-fork utensil he ate with—and the splint that fitted it to his hand, the leg-bag and the catheter and the stoma, his trousers with the zipper up the leg, his bulbous stomach, the single muscle in his shoulder, the scars of his many operations, the new pressure sores that already were festering on his backside from so long a time in the chair, his teeth, the bright caps that replaced them when his real teeth decalcified after the spinal break, his miniature arms and legs, the growing hump on his back, his hard celibacy and his broken neck. And the thought that he had, in this red and swirling landscape, was that they were not hateful things to gaze upon, and not symbolic of anything, but only real and worthy of his love. Twilah was there in all the redness, the long-lost girl with the freckles and the orange hair, who for so long had been only a symbol of everything Winston had missed in life and who now was only Twilah, a girl he never knew and could scarcely remember. It was a gentle red whirlwind that harmed no one. His father was there with a duckcall, his mother washing dewberries. The ambulance door slammed shut and the siren started up. Winston hoped he could make Harris understand.

35

God's Goodness: A Short Story

℘ Marjorie Kemper

First, last, and foremost, Ling Tan thought of herself as a Christian. So when Mrs. Sheriday said, "Tell me a little something about yourself," Ling didn't even draw breath before responding, "I am good Christian." And so saying, she sat up even straighter in her chair, like a star pupil providing the correct answer to a teacher.

But the employment counselor didn't smile. She didn't even look up. She went on regarding the papers on her desk and said, "Well, yes, I'm sure that you are. But what I meant was, tell me more about your work experience. I see that you were enrolled in a practical-nursing program at Long Beach Memorial Hospital but you didn't complete the course of study."

Ling ducked her head.

"Why was that?"

Ling said nothing.

"Why, exactly, did you drop out?"

Ling smiled and shrugged.

The other woman waited.

The silence got too big for Ling. Twisting her hands, she said, "Had late classes. Afraid to ride bus home at night."

"I see." Mrs. Sheriday looked back down at the papers. "Next time try taking morning classes, because you need more credits." She pointed her pen at Ling's thin résumé. "Your references are very good; I can see you're good with patients. But our doctors and care managers like to see more academic training. You still have time to register for some classes at Long Beach Community College."

Ling nodded.

"Even if you were just enrolled, I could list them."

"Next semester I enroll," Ling said, and smiled. Americans liked smiling, and Californians smiled all the time, so Ling made it a habit to smile constantly. She smiled when she was alone; she might even have smiled in her sleep.

As Ling got up to leave, Mrs. Sheriday said, "Check with me midweek— I might have something then. I see you've worked with children. I have a pediatric oncologist who is looking for somebody to live in and provide custodial care for a patient who is terminal. You wouldn't have any expenses, and you could save your wages for next school term."

Ling nodded, and in acknowledgment of the seriousness of this new topic, the mortal illness of a child, attempted to stop smiling. But this was not quite possible.

Back in her furnished room, two hours later, Ling drank three glasses of water. She drank the first one because she was thirsty from sitting on the bus-stop bench in the hot sun for an hour; she drank the second and third to trick her stomach into thinking she had fed it breakfast and lunch. She sat in a chair she had placed at the uncurtained window of her second-story room. It was spring, and in a yard beyond a shabby garage two plum trees—un-pruned for a generation—were struggling into bloom. Ling let her eyes rest on the white blossoms and took the time to thank God for the beauty he had created in every moment and in every place. Even now, even here. Wherever she looked she could see evidence of his goodness. And the flowering plums were beautiful—if Ling looked only at their canopies, if her eye didn't fol-low the scaling trunks down to the array of old paint cans and junk lumber nestled in the weeds beneath.

Ling took a deep breath and thanked God for his unceasing goodness to her—air in abundance, strong lungs to take it in, the flowering plums, even the water in her plastic glass. Ling sat in her chair and watched the plum trees until dusk fell and the blossoms melted into the darkness. Then, hav-ing no food and no money to buy it, she went to bed. In her neighborhood children played late; car alarms went on and off, seemingly at random; po-lice cars and ambulances wailed on their way to St. Mary's Hospital, a block away. Even after she'd pulled the shades down, the orange streetlights cast a hellish glow on the ceiling. Ling shut her eyes and prayed. She was deep in a prayer of thanksgiving for her many blessings when she fell asleep.

Ling called Mrs. Sheriday on Wednesday from a pay phone on the corner of her street. "Ling, I'm glad you called. I got a call from the doctor about that boy. I made a tentative appointment for you to go out and meet his mother, Mrs. Tipton. The parents are divorced."

Ling smiled furiously into the phone.

Martha Tipton, the sick boy's mother, opened the door to Ling Tan. While still in the vestibule, Mrs. Tipton said, "Oh, dear, you don't look very strong—you're shorter than Mike."

"Oh, very strong," Ling said. "Not big, not tall, but very strong. Used to working with children."

"Mike's sixteen. He doesn't weigh what he should, of course, but he's tall for his age."

Ling smiled. "Very strong," she repeated.

Mrs. Tipton led the way into the living room. "Well, if you say so. Mrs. Sheriday said you'd be bringing references. May I see them?"

Ling opened her purse and proffered the letters, and Mrs. Tipton sat down on the edge of the sofa to read them. Ling remained standing. The living room was sparsely furnished—a sofa, a piano, a bare coffee table. All of Mrs. Tipton's domestic efforts appeared to have gone into her yard and her plants. From the sidewalk Ling had already noticed, with approval, Mrs. Tipton's well-kept garden. Now Ling's eyes went to a row of African violets on a low windowsill—pink ones, white ones, purple ones—all blooming! Mrs. Tipton was a good steward.

"These are remarkable," Mrs. Tipton said, handing the letters back to Ling. "Let's go back to Mike's room and see if he's awake." When they got there, Mrs. Tipton stuck her head inside. "He's sleeping," she whispered, closing the door quietly.

"Will I sleep close by, so can hear boy if he call?" Ling asked.

Mrs. Tipton nodded and opened the next door—into a small room containing a bureau, a sewing machine, an ironing board, and a single bed. "I've cleared out the bureau for your things," she said.

The room had French doors. Outside, healthy ferns and fuchsias cascaded from hanging baskets, and nasturtiums bordered the brick walk. God's goodness, as well as Mrs. Tipton's fine stewardship, was much in evidence.

Ling transported her belongings—a green leatherette suitcase and a canvas satchel holding her Bible and her Bible-study books—on the bus later that afternoon. When she arrived, at six, Mike was asleep again, and Mrs. Tipton was preparing to leave for an appointment with her tax man.

"Mike's had his dinner," she said. "He usually eats at five-thirty. Just go in and introduce yourself when he wakes up. And when you do, give him the pills in this paper cup. I've told him about you, and he's expecting to meet you. If you should need me, the number is on the refrigerator, beside Doctor Mackenzie's."

After Mrs. Tipton had gone, Ling checked on Mike. She stood in the doorway to his room and studied her new charge for a long time. He was blond, pale, and tall, as his mother had said—or, more accurate in the circumstances, long. His bare arms were covered with a light blond down. Ling—who had been orphaned at eight and had survived typhus and thirty-two days in an open boat—could not accept the inevitability of the sleeping boy's death. Inevitability was a concept that ran contrary to her experience. That afternoon, while discussing Mike's illness with Mrs. Tipton, Ling had said that she would pray for a miracle for Mike. Mrs. Tipton's brow had furrowed, and she'd said that it was a little late in the day for that. Ling had quickly dropped the subject, but she could not drop the hope. To Ling, who regarded her own life as an unfolding miracle, miracles were a commonplace.

Later, when Ling heard Mike's dry little cough floating down the hall, she ran to his doorway and spoke quietly. "Mike, I Ling Tan. I here to help Mother take care of you until you get better." She smiled at the boy—who pushed himself higher on his pillows and studied her face. Ling went on, "Mother just go to see tax man. Back very soon."

"I don't know where you got your information, Ling Tan," Mike said severely, "but I'm not getting better. I'm in the process of getting worse."

"Naughty boy!" Ling exclaimed, laughing as she rushed forward into the room to tuck in a loose cover at the foot of his bed. "Now Ling here, you stop getting worse. Start getting better!"

"You could maybe benefit from a little chat with my oncologist," Mike said, taking a pillow from behind his back and pounding it into a new shape.

"I tell him thing or two. You hungry?"

"No."

"Mother make you little snack. Leave in refrigerator."

Ling went to the kitchen and came back with a bowl of sliced peaches. "Here," she said. "Look good. Eat peach. Give you energy to get better."

"Have you ever heard of white cells?"

"No."

"Lucky you."

Ling nodded. "Lucky all my life—but not luck really. *Grace.*" She sat down at the foot of Mike's bed. "Grace better than luck. You pray for grace, Mike. Not look nice to pray for luck."

Mike ate a peach slice. "I'll remember that," he said, and he picked up the TV remote from his bedside table. As the TV sprang to life, a sitcom audience screamed with laughter; Mike muted the TV. "I'd like to know what's so damn funny," he said.

Ling said, "Nothing that funny, don't think. I read in magazine, studio bring crazy people to TV shows in buses, to laugh like pack of monkeys."

"Hyenas," Mike corrected. "The expression is 'pack of hyenas.'"

Ling nodded. "Hyenas," she repeated. "Bring them from crazy house."

"That explains a lot," Mike said. He flipped through the channels until he found a rerun of *M*A*S*H*.

"Oh, like this program," Ling said enthusiastically. "Good doctors on this program. Funny."

"Not very realistic, though," Mike said. "I've yet to meet a doctor with even a rudimentary sense of humor."

Ling nodded brightly.

"Aren't you supposed to bring me my meds?"

Ling looked away from the TV, where Klinger was dressed like a woman. "Oh, I forget! I get them right now."

She handed Mike a glass of water and watched while he transferred six pills from the paper cup to his mouth and swallowed them. She said, "So many!"

"Yes, and they accomplish so little."

"But good for you—make you better."

Mike turned the TV back up. Ling returned to the foot of his bed. She sat sideways and turned her head to watch. "Klinger wear same dress as my auntie," she told Mike, and giggled.

Mike snorted. "I hope it looked better on her."

"Didn't," Ling said with a laugh. "Auntie not look good, but Auntie good inside." Ling tapped her breast. "Here."

She gazed around Mike's room. It had a wall of bookshelves, and a desk and chair by the window. A picture of Mike's parents sat on the bureau, taken when they were much younger. They were holding hands. Ling turned away; photos made her nervous. They were always of things that were over with, gone—a moment, a smile, a person, sometimes a whole country. A poster of an old man with scraggly hair was on the back of Mike's door. The man was sticking his tongue out. Why did Mike have a picture of a crazy person on his door? "Who is that?" she asked cautiously, in case it was a relative.

"Einstein."

Ling smiled and nodded.

"He was a physicist," Mike said. "A genius," he added for Ling's benefit, because she still looked blank. "You've heard of E equals MC squared?"

Ling smiled and nodded. "Are you genius too? Have so many books!"

"I'm smart, but possibly not a genius."

"How come he make that face?"

"Why not?"

"I try go to college, learn more, but my English not very good," Ling confided. "I quit before bad grades get on permanent record." She had never told this to anyone before.

"Your English isn't so bad," Mike said. "Considering."

"Maybe you help me—tell me when I using wrong word."

"It would have to be a crash course. My mother must have told you I'm on my way out. We're talking months here, Ling Tan." Mike ran through the channels with the remote. "Two, maybe three." He clicked the set off. "Tops."

"Mother can't know everything. Doctors either. I wait and see."

"An empiricist in our midst," Mike said.

"A what?"

"An empiricist is someone who draws conclusions from the evidence."

"Not Empiricist—Christian. Believe in God's goodness. In miracles."

"That's what it would take."

Ling nodded smartly. "Already praying. Start without you. You see. God is good. He bless us every day."

"You could have fooled me," Mike said.

Ling quickly fit herself into the routine of the Tipton household. Fitting in was what she did best; it was her special gift. She could be quiet, as she had been when her family had hidden from the soldiers in the forest. She could make herself small, as she had in the boat. If necessary, she could even push herself forward and talk fast and loud, as she had in the refugee camp. With Mike she was cheerful as a rule. Early on they developed a vaudeville routine of sorts, with Mike playing Baby Curmudgeon to her Cheerful Naif.

With Mrs. Tipton, Ling was careful to be quiet and pleasant. Mrs. Tipton's nerves were ragged, and she frequently burst into tears in the course of ordinary conversations. Not wanting Mike to see her cry, she spent a lot of time outside, working in her garden. She came into her son's room at frequent intervals, but rarely stayed long. Usually she rushed off, saying she needed to check on something—just seconds before bursting into tears.

When Mr. Tipton came over, Ling endeavored to make herself invisible. Though she suspected that Mr. Tipton was every bit as sad as his ex-wife, he seemed more angry than sad. He seemed to be angry all the time, at everything and everyone except Mike.

When Ling first met him, she recognized him right away from the photo in his son's room. Unlike poor Mrs. Tipton, Mr. Tipton looked the same as in Mike's photo. When Ling opened the door to him, she said, "Oh! Mike's father! He will be so happy to see you."

"Where's Martha?"

"Go to market. Back soon. I'm Ling Tan."

When she heard Mrs. Tipton's car in the driveway, Ling went out to help carry the groceries. "Mr. Tipton here with Mike," she said. Ling put away the groceries while Mrs. Tipton went back to Mike's room.

Shortly thereafter Mr. Tipton came out to the kitchen. He looked very angry. "Mike tells me you're praying for him."

Ling felt herself accused, and ducked her head. "Yes," she admitted.

"Well, naturally you're free to pray day and night, but I'd appreciate your not talking to Mike about it. Or about miracles. We've spent two years choking on hope around here; hope is ancient history. I appreciate your intentions, but the last thing we need is a latecomer peddling miracles."

Mr. Tipton had spoken quickly and softly, and though Ling had certainly gotten the sense of what he'd said, she'd missed some of the words. What, for instance, did "peddling" mean? Looking down at the floor, she said, "Just try to keep up boy's spirits."

Every morning, when she brought in Mike's breakfast and pills, she opened his drapes and delivered her line: "Look, Mikey! God make another beautiful day just for you. He expect you to *look* at it."

His line was "Close the damn drapes. It's too bright."

"Too bright for moles, maybe," Ling always responded. "You not mole. You boy."

One morning when Ling opened the drapes she saw Mike's mother kneeling in the garden. "Look, Mikey, Mother planting new flowers for you to see out window. Wave at her." Mike rolled his eyes, but he waved. His mother was kneeling in the dirt, transferring pansies from flats into a flower bed around the deodar tree in the side yard. Surprised, she smiled and waved back.

"Your mother best gardener I know," Ling observed. "She love her plants. They feel it and grow big for her."

"She loves me, too, but this is as big as I'm getting."

"You plenty big already," Ling said. "Bigger than me."

"What *is* this?" Mike asked when Ling lifted the lid from a bowl on his breakfast tray.

"Oatmeal."

"I don't like oatmeal."

"Oatmeal good for you. You eat, then maybe I bring something you like."

"Whose bright idea is this?"

"My idea. I read in magazine when we at Doctor Mackenzie's office, oatmeal cleanse the blood."

"Jesus, Ling, get a clue."

"Won't hurt you to eat little bowl of oatmeal," Ling said.

☙

Because Mrs. Tipton took pills and slept soundly, one of Ling's jobs was to listen for Mike during the night. If he needed her, he knocked on their shared wall. After helping him to the bathroom, or getting him something to drink or a pill or—on a bad night—a shot, or rubbing his foot when he had a cramp, Ling kept him company until he was able to sleep again. One night, curled up like a cat at the foot of Mike's bed, Ling asked, "You want to watch TV? Maybe *M*A*S*H* on." It usually was.

"Not really. Has my dad bawled you out about this miracle deal?"

"Not know 'bawled out.'"

"Did he yell at you?"

"Not yell," Ling said. "Father worried for you. Not want me upset you."

"I was afraid of that. I want you to know I didn't complain about you. I only mentioned it to him because I thought he'd get a kick out of it. I was a little off the mark there. Shows you how well I know dear old Dad. Anyway, I hope he didn't hurt your feelings."

"Not hurt my feelings. Don't need Father's permission to pray. Don't need permission for miracle either."

"I wouldn't think so."

"Father love you very much. Tell me getting special doctor for you." Mr. Tipton had informed Ling and Mrs. Tipton that he'd arranged for a psychiatrist who worked with terminally ill children and adolescents to visit Mike.

"You mean the shrink?"

Ling smiled and shook her head to indicate that she didn't know the word.

"S-H-R-I-N-K—that's another word for a head doctor. One of the high priests of humanism."

"Ah," Ling said. "Father's priest?"

Mike snorted. "Close enough. He's supposed to make me feel better about dying."

"He can do that?"

"We shall see." Mike closed his eyes.

"You want me read to you?"

"Sure."

"Same book Father read this afternoon?" Father and son were reading Hegel. Ling had no idea what it was about; all she knew was that it had more hard words than the Bible and no story at all.

"Not this time of night. You pick something."

Ling ran to her room and came back with her Bible. "I read to you from *my* book." Laughing, she held it up for Mike to see.

"Oh, Dad would love this!"

"He say not talk about miracle. Didn't say about *Bible*."

"True," Mike said. "I know—read the Book of Job. Let's get a standard of comparison."

"Oh, Job *sad* story."

"My favorite kind."

But about fifteen minutes into Job's travails Mike's pain pill took effect, and he fell asleep. Ling stopped reading. She sat very still until she was certain that the boy was sleeping soundly, and then she moved to the desk chair. Ling tried to go on reading (she'd left off where Job said, "Wearisome nights are appointed to me"), but the light from the little bedside lamp was too distant to read by, so she shut the book and put her head down on the desk. The miracle she'd been praying for since arriving at the Tiptons' was nowhere in sight, and even Ling, always optimistic, always on the lookout for a blessing, understood that they were running low on time. Mike kept getting thinner, despite the nice meals his mother prepared, meals that Ling spent hours coaxing the boy to eat. Fortunately, she'd been telling Mrs. Tipton the truth when she'd said that she was strong, because nowadays she more carried than walked Mike to the bathroom. They had stopped going downtown to the medical building to see his oncologist. Now Dr. Mackenzie came to the house, rushing in and staying only long enough to rationalize his big bill and to cast a pall over everyone's spirits. Mike's cough had grown worse. At last count nine pills were in the paper cup after dinner, and, most ominous, syringes of pain medicine were now kept in the refrigerator for the relief of Mike's severe headaches, which came on without warning. All in all, Ling had a lot to pray for and about; her head cradled in her thin arms, she was still praying when the sun came up.

The new doctor, Dr. Hanson, the shrink, came to the house three afternoons a week. On his first visit, every time Mike had said anything, Dr. Hanson had responded, "How does that make you feel, Mike?"

"Like death warmed over," Mike had said, trying to fluster him. Or "Makes me want to die," or "Scares me to death." Ling and Mike had exchanged conspiratorial glances, and Ling had laughed behind her hand.

But Dr. Hanson proved to be such a nice young man that teasing him wasn't much fun. In fact, after he'd been coming for a couple of weeks, Mike told Ling that he felt sorry for Dr. Hanson.

"Why sorry for him?" she snapped. "You the sick one."

"Yeah, but he's so damn hopeful, you know?"

"Bible say hope a virtue. Have to hope."

"For what?"

Ling shrugged. "Just hope." She had begun to resent this particular injunction.

"You're saying that this mandatory hope has no object?"

Ling thought for a minute and said, "Hope is to prop open door, so good things can come in. Maybe when you not looking."

"I see. Hope as a metaphysical doorstop. Good one, Ling. Well, anyway, at least Doctor Hanson *talks*. Doctor Mackenzie hasn't said two personal words to me in weeks."

"He lose interest in us, I think."

"I know. I shouldn't have played so hard to get. And probably I should have eaten more *oatmeal*. It's abundantly clear that I've no one to blame for all this but myself."

Ling looked at the floor. She'd thrown the box of oatmeal in the garbage a week before. "Maybe should invite some boys, Mikey, come talk to you. You have some nice friends own age?"

"Not really. Do you?"

"Not really," Ling admitted. "We each other's friend now, I think."

"Works for me."

&

As Mike grew worse, the room filled with sickroom apparatus—first a walker, then a commode, and finally, after a series of consecutive bad nights, a rollaway bed for Ling. While Mike slept, Ling went through the Book of Job, which had become a favorite of Mike's, with a fine-tooth comb, hoping to find some consolation. After God had let the Devil have his way with Job, after Job had brought credit on him, God took him back. The Bible even said that afterward God gave Job new sons and daughters, new cattle and sheep. And, Ling supposed, cattle were cattle, and one cow was as good as another, but children were not cattle. Children had souls. You could not replace one with another. So where was the comfort in all this?

But Mike read Job over and over. He memorized great hunks of it, and insisted on reading his favorite bits aloud to Ling. Sometimes he stopped mid-sentence and laughed.

"I'm in your debt for suggesting this, Ling."

"No problem," Ling said. "God's word count for something in this world, but I not go to college, and not a genius, so I not always sure what."

"Yes you are," Mike said.

Ling shook her head.

"You believe in God's goodness still, don't you?"

Ling turned her back on Mike and looked out the window.

"You do, don't you, Ling?"

"Have to believe in that when I look at God's big world," Ling said.

"There you go," Mike said. "The world is very, very big. It stands to reason that it's beyond our understanding, yes?"

"Yes," Ling whispered. "But used to understand."

"And now you don't. You see, you've learned something already."

"What I am learning?"

"That there's more to heaven and earth than oatmeal and a positive attitude. More than Ling Tan was born knowing. Humility—not to put too fine a point on it."

Humility was a hard lesson, worse than English grammar, and Ling missed her old, blithe assurance as keenly as she might have missed a beloved pet. But she believed what she had told Mikey about hope—that you could use it to prop open a door so that something good might come in. So she hoped. And waited. And prayed for something good to slip through their open door. Maybe at night, while they slept.

Dr. Hanson was an even bigger smiler than Ling—who these days had to remind herself to smile, and who thought that the young doctor overdid it.

"Doctor Hanson always so cheerful," Ling remarked one day, while she folded laundry on Mike's bed. She didn't mean it as a compliment.

"And why not?" Mike asked. "He's not the one who's dying. Though I don't know why he doesn't get right on it, since he sees it as such a gigantic opportunity for what he calls 'personal growth.'"

Ling giggled. "I think he already grow big *enough*." The doctor was a little on the plump side.

Mike laughed. "When he was here yesterday, I quoted some Job at him—'Thine hands have made me and fashioned me together round about; yet thou dost destroy me.' I wanted his take on that."

"What did he say?"

"He said, 'Beautiful, beautiful!' With this huge, ecstatic smile plastered on that big round face of his."

"How did that make you feel?" Ling said, joking.

"Like I'd been dead three days," Mike shot back.

"Maybe Job beautiful if not about *you*," Ling said, smoothing a pillowcase. She almost wished she hadn't introduced Mikey to the Bible. She'd certainly had it with Job and his comforters—even Job's God, whom she'd just barely contrived to keep separate from her own. These days, when she had the time and the energy to read, she stuck strictly to the Psalms and the Gospels. But Mike liked Job almost as much as he liked Einstein. Certainly more than Mr. Tipton at this point in the proceedings liked Hegel. Mike had told his mother that Job was his favorite book—which caused Mrs. Tipton to run out of the room in tears, and which she wisely did not pass on to her ex-husband. When Ling brought in Mike's breakfast, he always quoted, in a rising falsetto, "Or is there *any* taste in the white of an egg?"

Folding towels, Ling said, "I think Doctor Hanson look better if he grow beard. Then his face not seem so wide."

"I'll tell him."

"No, Mikey! Then he know we notice his face fat." Piling the folded laundry back in the basket, Ling confessed, "Mikey, worried about miracle. Afraid prayers aren't getting through."

"Sure they are," Mike said. "It's the answers that seem to be snagged up."

"Same thing," Ling said.

"Not necessarily."

Ling nodded. "Study guide say God answer prayers, but his answer not always one we want. No, I say it wrong: it say, maybe not answer we *expect*."

"Ah, the element of surprise. One of his favorite devices. As we've learned."

Ling took a deep breath and tried to smile at Mike's little joke. "Not giving up, Mikey. I keep praying. Promise."

"Everyone should have a hobby," Mike said, "to quote the estimable Doctor Hanson." He flipped on the TV.

Dr. Hanson had asked Mike what his hobbies were, and Mike had said that just lately his hobby was dying.

Undeterred, Dr. Hanson had said, "That's more of a full-time job, isn't it? I'm talking recreation. Do you play chess?"

After that Dr. Hanson and Mike played chess. Mike consistently beat him. But instead of saying "Checkmate," Mike would say, "How does that make you feel?"

"Beat," Dr. Hanson would reply. "Walloped."

"You don't think he's letting me win, do you?" Mike asked Ling later that week. He was having one of what he and Ling were calling his "bad days." He'd had a solid week of them. The smell of Dr. Hanson's after-shave still lingered in the room. Even his after-shave, Ling had protested to Mike, was cheerful.

"Doctor Hanson can't beat genius, Mikey."

"I may not be a genius, Ling. It's impossible at this point to tell for sure."

"Close. Maybe not like old Uncle." Ling pointed at the Einstein poster. "But you not old like him either. Smarter than Doctor Hanson for sure! What he thinking? *Smiling* every minute at boy supposed to be dying!"

"You should talk."

"I know. Used to smile like hyena."

"Monkey! No, monkeys *grin*, don't they? Hyenas laugh. *Lings* smile."

"Ling not so much smiling now. Only when something to smile about. You notice?"

"Actually, I've been meaning to talk to you about that. I think it's time to paste a big old smile on your face and leave it there, because we're definitely running out of reasons. Anyway, on you a smile has always looked good."

Ling smiled. It was an effort.

A month later Dr. Hanson stopped smiling. Mike was in a coma. Still Dr. Hanson came at his appointed times and sat beside Mike's bed and held the boy's hand—now studded like a clove orange with IVs. Dr. Mackenzie came every day, and a registered nurse came morning and evening. Mr. and Mrs. Tipton took turns sitting in Mike's room—Mrs. Tipton crying freely now, her hands clasped in her lap; Mr. Tipton staring at an open book, the pages of which he rarely turned. Ling sat out of the way, in Mike's desk chair, which she had pulled over to the window so that she could look out at Mrs. Tipton's garden.

On the night before he'd slipped into the coma, Ling and Mike had tried to watch *M*A*S*H*, but Mike had a terrible headache, and the light from the TV hurt his eyes. Ling had turned it off.

"We see that one already," she said briskly. By then they'd seen them all. "That one sad anyway. Even Hawkeye cry." Mike, eyes shut, nodded. Ling gave him his pain shot and rubbed his temples with a Chinese herbal lotion that her auntie had used for migraines.

"My God, what is this stuff?" Mike protested. "It smells like a bog!"

"All natural," Ling assured him. "Very good for headache. Cleanse the blood. Good for bad nerves."

"I can't *believe* you're still trying to cleanse this treacherous blood of mine! However," Mike conceded, "my nerves could not be worse."

"Auntie swear by it," Ling said. She smoothed his thin hair back, rubbing his forehead.

Mike looked up into her eyes. "You know where we made our mistake, don't you?"

Ling shook her head.

"Praying for grace instead of luck. We tipped our hand. We indicated we were willing to *settle*."

Ling bit her lower lip and didn't answer.

"Come on, Ling. 'How does that make you feel?'"

Ling giggled weakly. "Don't," she said. "Too tired to joke."

It was three in the morning. The only noise in the house was the refrigerator humming in the kitchen. Mike closed his eyes and quoted: "God thundereth marvelously with his voice; great things doeth he, which we cannot comprehend."

"That not God, that the refrigerator."

"Maybe, maybe not. You'll admit that the universe, or God—whatever you like to call it—*does* stuff we don't get. Hegel didn't get it. I'm not even sure Einstein got it."

"He get it. That's why he stick tongue out."

Mike snorted.

Ling took a long breath. She put the cap back on the bottle of Auntie's lotion and said, "Maybe God blessing us this moment, and we not knowing it."

"Thanks for trying, Ling, but that may be the single most depressing thing you've said to me."

"Not depressing, Mikey. I only mean he bless me with you and he bless you with me."

❧

The morning after Mike died, after she'd packed and before she left Mrs. Tipton's house forever, Ling went into Mike's room. She had made up the empty bed the night before. Now she went to the window and pulled back the drapes.

"God make another beautiful day, Mikey," she said. Then, after blowing her nose and replacing the ragged Kleenex in the pocket of her sweater, she added, "But this one not for you."

Ling stood staring out Mike's window. The dew was still on the grass; though Mrs. Tipton lay sedated in her bed, her lawn shone brightly in the morning light. The little faces of her pansies were turned up to the sun. The beauty of the flowers, and the sunshine they sought, were, Ling still believed, firm and undeniable evidence of God's goodness. Even here and even now. But this knowledge no longer lifted her up. She placed the palm of her hand on Mikey's empty bed and briefly bowed her head.

When she turned to go, her gaze met Einstein's. She had noticed a month before that except for the rude face he was making, Mikey's old scientist looked a lot like the illustrations of God the Father in her Bible-study guide. She had shown Mikey, who had thought this a hilarious coincidence. Now, her hand on the doorknob, Ling looked into the old face that had looked down on them for months, silently regarding everything they had done and suffered.

"Good-bye, Mr. Genius," she said softly. Then, before she sailed out the door, and in recognition, or solidarity, or maybe just farewell, Ling stuck out her little pink tongue.

Resources

The following is a selected list of resources in two main categories, medical humanities and family caregiving. Each item has references and links to other resources.

MEDICAL HUMANITIES

WEBSITES

www.narrativemedicine.org   The website of the Program in Narrative Medicine at the College of Physicians and Surgeons at Columbia University, directed by Rita Charon, MD, has extensive resources in this growing field. There are bibliographies, links to other university programs, specialized sites, and other resources.

litmed.med.nyu.edu   The New York University Medical School's database in medical humanities has annotated references to art, literature, and performing arts. It is frequently updated.

www.narrativemedicinenetwork.org   The International Network of Narrative Medicine is a joint effort of King's College, London, and the Program in Narrative Medicine, Columbia University.

BOOKS

Nell Casey, *An Uncertain Inheritance: Writers on Caring for Family* (New York: Morrow, 2007).

Rita Charon, *Narrative Medicine: Honoring the Stories of Illness* (New York: Oxford University Press, 2008).

Arthur Frank, *The Wounded Storyteller: Body, Illness, and Ethics*, 2nd edition (Chicago: University of Chicago Press, 2013).

Arthur Kleinman, *The Illness Narratives: Suffering, Healing, and the Human Condition* (New York: Basic Books, 1989).

Suzanne Poirier and Lioness Ayres, eds. *Stories of Family Caregivers: Reconsiderations of Theory, Literature, and Life* (Indianapolis: Center Nursing Publishing, 2002).

FAMILY CAREGIVING

WEBSITES

www.aarp.org/home-family/caregiving The AARP Caregiving Resource Center has information about AARP programs, blogs, columns by experts, and other information.

www.alz.org The Alzheimer's Association website is a major resource for family caregivers for people with Alzheimer's and other dementias. It has research reports, support for family caregivers, guides to local chapters, and other resources.

www.caregiver.org Family Caregiver Alliance's website has a wide range of materials, including research reports, caregiving information and advice, policy briefs, and other features.

www.medicare.gov/campaigns/caregiver/caregiver.html The Medicare website has information about benefits and other government resources.

www.nextstepincare.org The United Hospital Fund's Next Step in Care website has an extensive list of easy-to-use guides for family caregivers navigating transitions in health care settings. The guides are free and available in English, Spanish, Chinese, and Russian. There are also guides for health care providers working with family caregivers. The Links and Resources section suggests federal, state, and local resources for further information, as well as links to disease organizations.

newoldage.blogs.nytimes.com The *New York Times* New Old Age blog has timely posts by Paula Span, Judith Graham, and others on topics related to family caregiving including financial matters, relationships, practical tips, and many other subjects.

www.wellspouse.org The Well Spouse Association website has stories from well spouses, event announcements, and other information for this group of caregivers.

BOOKS

American Red Cross, *Family Caregiving* (Yardley, PA: StayWell, 2007).
> A book in the American Red Cross Safety series, this spiral-bound book has practical directions for taking care of a sick or disabled person at home. There is an accompanying DVD.

Jane Gross, *A Bittersweet Season: Caring for Our Aging Parents—and Ourselves* (New York: Knopf, 2011).
> Part memoir, part guide through the world of hospitals, nursing homes, and finances, written by a former *New York Times* reporter.

Barry Jacobs, *The Emotional Survival Guide for Caregivers: Looking after Yourself and Your Family While Helping an Aging Parent* (New York: Guilford Press, 2006).
> Written by a clinical psychologist, this book has useful advice on coping with the emotional strain of caregiving.

Carol Levine, ed., *Always On Call: When Illness Turns Families into Caregivers*, 2nd edition (Nashville: Vanderbilt University Press, 2004).
> A section with personal narratives is followed by chapters on employment, public policy, the emotional impact of caregiving, and other topics.

Nancy L. Mace and Peter V. Rabins, *The 36-Hour Day: A Family Guide to Caring for Persons with Alzheimer Disease, Related Dementing Illnesses, and Memory Loss in Later Life*, 4th edition (Baltimore: Johns Hopkins University Press, 2006).
> This classic guide was revised in 2006 for its twenty-fifth anniversary.

Gail Sheehy, *Passages in Caregiving: Turning Chaos into Confidence* (New York: William Morrow, 2010).
> Sheehy, a well-known writer, describes her experiences over the many years she cared for her husband who had cancer.

Paula Span, *When the Time Comes: Families with Aging Parents Share Their Struggles and Solutions* (New York: Springboard Press, 2009).
> Span is a journalist who interviewed several families for this helpful book.

Contributors

Dick Allen is a poet whose numerous poetry collections include *Present Vanish: Poems* (2008) and *Ode to the Cold War: Poems New and Selected* (1997). Until his retirement he was Director of Creative Writing and Charles A. Dana Endowed Chair Professor at the University of Bridgeport (CT). In 2010 he was named poet laureate of Connecticut and will serve in that position through 2015.

Chana Bloch is a poet and translator of works in Hebrew. Her collections of poems are *The Secrets of the Tribe* (1981), *The Past Keeps Changing* (1992), *Mrs. Dumpty* (1998), and *Blood Honey* (2009). She is Professor Emerita of English Literature and Creative Writing at Mills College.

Anne Brashler was a short story writer and poet. Her stories are collected in *Getting Jesus in the Mood* (1991) and her poems in *The Talking Poems* (1994). She was one of two artists who conducted a residency at Bell Elementary School in Chicago in 1990 through the Illinois Arts Council's Arts-in-Education Artist Residency Program. Brashler died in 2013.

Rosellen Brown has written novels, short stories, and poetry. Among her novels are *Tender Mercies* (1978), *Civil Wars* (1984), and *Half a Heart* (2000). Her novel *Before and After* (1992) was made into a film of the same name in 1996. A collection of stories, *Street Games*, was published in 1991. She teaches in the MFA Writing Program at the School of the Art Institute in Chicago.

Ethan Canin is a writer and physician. Among his novels are *America, America* (2008), and *For Kings and Planets* (2010). His story collections include *Emperor of the Air* (1998) and *The Palace Thief* (1994). He is on the faculty of the Iowa Writers Workshop at the University of Iowa.

Raymond Carver was a major American short-story writer and poet. His most famous story is "What We Talk About When We Talk About Love." The poem in this volume is from his collection *Ultramarine*, published in 1986. Carver died in 1988.

Eugenia Collier is an African-American writer and educator. She taught English at colleges and universities in the Baltimore-Washington area until her retirement in 1996. With Richard A. Long, she co-edited

Afro-American Writing (1992), and she is the author of *Breeder and Other Stories* (1993). In 2010 she published a novel, *Beyond the Crossroads*.

Sarah Day has published several collections of poems, most recently *Grass Notes* (2009). Her poems have been set to music by British composer Anthony Gilbert. She was poetry editor of *Island Magazine* for seven years, teaches English and Creative Writing, and has been a council member of the Literature Board of the Australia. She lives in Hobart, Tasmania.

James Dickey was a poet from Georgia who served in the US Air Force in World War II. From 1996–1998 he was the Poetry Consultant to the Library of Congress, a position that later became Poet Laureate. His best-selling novel *Deliverance* (1970) was made into a movie. Among his poetry collections are *Buckdancer's Choice* (1965) and *The Whole Motion: Collected Poems 1945–1992* (1992). Dickey died in 1997.

Mark Doty is a poet and Professor/Writer in Residence at Rutgers University. His book *Fire to Fire: New and Selected Poems* won the National Book Award for Poetry in 2008. He has published eight books of poems and four volumes of nonfiction prose. His most recent work is *A Swarm, A Flock, A Host: A Compendium of Creatures* (2013), an illustrated bestiary with Darren Waterston.

Tereze Glück is the author of *May You Live in Interesting Times* (1995), a collection of stories. She is now a goldsmith and jewelry designer in New York.

Allegra Goodman is a novelist and short-story writer who grew up in Hawaii and now lives in Cambridge, MA. Her novels include *The Family Markowitz* (1996), *Kaaterskill Falls* (1998), *Paradise Park* (2001), and *Intuition* (2006). Her most recent novel is *The Cookbook Collector* (2010). She has also written a science fiction book for young readers, *The Other Side of the Island* (2008).

Mary Gordon has written novels, short stories, memoirs, and essays about religion. Among her novels are *Final Payment* (1978), *The Other Side* (1989), *Pearl* (2005), and *The Love of My Youth* (2011). Her story collections include *Temporary Shelter* (1987) and *The Stories of Mary Gordon* (2006). Her memoirs include *The Shadow Man: A Daughter Searches for her Father* (1996) and *Circling My Mother* (2007). She is a professor of English at Barnard College.

Rachel Hadas is a poet, professor, essayist, and translator. She published a memoir about her husband's illness, *Strange Relation*, in 2011. Her most recent book of poems, *The Golden Road*, was published in 2012. She teaches in the English Department of the Newark campus of Rutgers University.

Donald Hall is a poet and essayist who has published fifteen books of poetry, most recently *White Apples and Taste of Stone: Selected Poems 1946–2006* (2007), *The Painted Bed* (2002), and *Without: Poems* (1998), which was published on the third anniversary of his wife Jane Kenyon's death from leukemia. In 2005 he published a memoir *The Best Day the Worst Day: Life with Jane Kenyon*. Hall was Poet Laureate of the United States from 2006–2007.

Amy Hanridge is an Arizona-based freelance writer whose stories have been published in several literary journals. She is also an adjunct online writing instructor and is working on a novel.

Ann Harleman is the author of the short story collections *Thoreau's Laundry* (2007) and *Happiness* (1994) and the novels *The Year She Disappeared* (2008) and *Bitter Lake* (1996). She is on the faculties of Brown University and the Rhode Island School of Design, where she teaches fiction writing to visual artists.

Tony Hoagland is a poet whose collections include *What Narcissism Means to Me* (2003), *Donkey Gospel* (1998), and *Sweet Ruin* (1992). His most recent collection is *Unincorporated Persons in the Late Honda Dynasty: Poems* (2010). He teaches in the creative writing program at the University of Houston and in the MFA program at Warren Wilson College.

Gish Jen (a pen name) is a writer whose parents emigrated from China in the 1940s. Her novels include *Mona in the Promised Land* (1997), *The Love Wife* (2005), and *Typical American* (2008). She published a collection of stories, *Who's Irish?*, in 2000. "The Third Dumpster" was included in *The Best American Short Stories 2013*.

Ha Jin (a pen name) left his native China in 1985 to attend American universities. He is the author of five novels including *Waiting* (1999), *A Free Life* (2007), and *Nanjing Requiem* (2011); four story collections including *The Bridegroom* (2000) and *A Good Fall* (2009); and three books of poetry. He is a professor of English at Boston University.

Marjorie Kemper is the author of the novel *Until That Good Day* (2003), loosely based on her family history of a traveling salesman who passed as a white man in Louisiana. Her published short stories have not been collected. She died in 2009.

Jane Kenyon was a poet whose works looked inward at her continuing efforts to overcome depression and outward at the domestic life in rural New England she shared with her husband Donald Hall. She published four volumes of poetry before she died in 1995: *From Room to Room* (1978); *The Little Boat* (1986); *Let Evening Come* (1990); and *Otherwise: New and Selected Poems* (1993). Her translations of the poems of Anna Akhmatova along with some essays and newspaper columns were published in *A Hundred White Daffodils* (1999).

Li-Young Lee is an American poet born in Indonesia of Chinese parents. His father was imprisoned as a political prisoner for a year and the family fled in 1959, when Lee was two years old. They arrived in America in 1964. *Rose*

(1986) was his first book of poetry. His most recent collection is *Behind My Eyes: Poems* (2009). He has also published *The Winged Seed: A Remembrance* (1995) and, with Earl G. Ingersoll, *Breaking the Alabaster Jar: Conversations with Li-Young Lee* (2006).

David Mason is a poet whose collections include *The Buried Houses* (1991) and *The Country I Remember* (1996). He is coeditor of four poetry anthologies and codirects the creative writing program at Colorado College.

W. S. Merwin has written over fifty books of poems and translations. They include *Migration: New and Selected Poems* (2005) and *The Shadow of Sirius* (2008). His most recent publication is *Selected Translations* (2013). He was US Poet Laureate from 2010 to 2011. He lives in Hawaii where he is actively involved in saving the island's rainforests.

Rick Moody is the author of the novels *Garden State* (1992), *The Ice Storm* (1994), and *Purple America* (1997), from which the selection in this volume is taken. He has also written two collections of short fiction: *The Ring of Brightest Angels Around Heaven* (1995) and *Demonology* (2001), as well as novellas and essays.

Lorrie Moore is the author of several novels, including *Who Will Run the Frog Hospital?* (1994) and *A Gate at the Stairs* (2009), and several story collections including *Self-Help* (1985), *Birds of America* (1998), and *The Collected Stories* (2008). She is a professor of English and taught creative writing at the University of Wisconsin-Madison. She is the Gertrude Conway Vanderbilt Professor of English at Vanderbilt University

Alice Munro is a Canadian writer who has published twelve collections of stories and two volumes of selected stories, as well as a novel, *Lives of Girls and Women* (1971). Her story collections include *Hateship, Friendship, Courtship, Loveship, Marriage* (2001), *Too Much Happiness* (2009), and *Dear Life: Stories* (2013). Alice Munro was awarded the Nobel Prize in Literature in 2013.

Lewis Nordan wrote stories and novels set in his native Mississippi. Among his short story collections are *Welcome to the Arrow-Catcher Fair* (1983) and *The All-Girl Football Team* (1986). His novels include *Wolf Whistle* (1993), based on the Emmett Till murder, and *The Sharpshooter Blues* (1995). In 2000 he published *Boy with Loaded Gun*, a "fictional memoir." He taught creative writing at the University of Pittsburgh until his retirement. He died in 2012.

Julie Otsuka has published two novels, *When the Emperor was Divine* (2002) and *The Buddha in the Attic* (2011). Her work reflects her Japanese-American family background, including their internment in World War II in a camp in Utah.

Robert Pinsky is a poet, essayist, critic, and translator. From 2007 to 2010 he was Poet Laureate of the United States. He has published numerous collections of poems, the most recent of which is *Selected Poems* (2011). With Maggie Dietz, he co-edited *America's Favorite Poems: The Favorite Poem Project Anthology* (1999). His translations include Dante's *Inferno* and works by Czeslaw Milosz.

C. K. Williams is a poet and translator. His collections include *Collected Poems* (2006), *Wait* (2010), and *Writers Writing Dying* (2012). He has written a memoir, *Misgivings* (2000), and has translated Sophocles and Europides.

Fran Pokras Yariv is the author of the novels *Learning* (2010) and *Last Exit* (2001). She and her sister Barbara Pokras published *Feeding Mrs. Moskowitz and The Caregiver: Two Stories*, from which the selection in this volume is taken, in 2010.

ABOUT THE EDITOR

Carol Levine directs the United Hospital Fund's Families and Health Care Project, which focuses on developing partnerships between health care professionals and family caregivers. She is a former editor of the *Hastings Center Report*, a journal devoted to medical ethics, and is now a Hastings Center Fellow. In 1993 she was awarded a MacArthur Foundation Fellowship for her work in AIDS policy and ethics. She edited *Always On Call: When Illness Turns Families into Caregivers*, 2nd edition (2004), and with Thomas H. Murray, co-edited *The Cultures of Caregiving: Conflict and Common Ground among Families, Health Professionals and Policy Maker* (2004). Her articles have been published in the *New England Journal of Medicine*, *Journal of the American Medical Association*, and other professional journals, as well as in *The New York Times* and other media. She has a BA in history from Cornell University, where she also studied Russian language and literature (with Vladimir Nabokov), and an MA from Columbia University in Public Law and Government.